Sonda Kammoun
Mona Rekik

Optical coherence tomography angiography

Sonda Kammoun
Mona Rekik

Optical coherence tomography angiography

in chorioretinal vascular pathologies

ScienciaScripts

Imprint
Any brand names and product names mentioned in this book are subject to trademark, brand or patent protection and are trademarks or registered trademarks of their respective holders. The use of brand names, product names, common names, trade names, product descriptions etc. even without a particular marking in this work is in no way to be construed to mean that such names may be regarded as unrestricted in respect of trademark and brand protection legislation and could thus be used by anyone.

Cover image: www.ingimage.com

This book is a translation from the original published under ISBN 978-620-6-72212-0.

Publisher:
Sciencia Scripts
is a trademark of
Dodo Books Indian Ocean Ltd. and OmniScriptum S.R.L publishing group

120 High Road, East Finchley, London, N2 9ED, United Kingdom
Str. Armeneasca 28/1, office 1, Chisinau MD-2012, Republic of Moldova, Europe
Printed at: see last page
ISBN: 978-620-8-27605-8

Table of contents

1. GENERAL INTRODUCTION

Retinal and choroidal imaging has long relied on the analysis of fluorescein angiography (FA) and indocyanine green infrared (ICGA). However, it turned out that these techniques do not show the retinal and/or choroidal structure, but only reveal the vascular content.

The advent of optical coherence tomography (OCT) has revolutionized ocular imaging. This technique, which provides histological sections of the retina, has become an essential tool in the diagnosis and treatment of posterior segment pathologies. Today, spectral domain OCT (SD-OCT) enables fine visualization of chorio-retinal micro-architectural details (1). It provides a clear view of the nerve retina, verifying photoreceptor integrity and reliably quantifying total retinal thickness, ganglion cell thickness, optic fiber thickness and choroidal thickness.

OCT-angiography (OCTA) is a new non-invasive imaging technique for retinal microvascularization, introduced in 2014 by the American company Optvue (2). Its principle is based on combining en face OCT imaging with the detection of movements within chorio-retinal vascular structures, from rapidly repeated B-scan OCT slices and thanks to "decorrelation" of the amplitude or phase of the signal obtained (3). Based on all the OCT B-scan sections acquired, the various software programs enable 3D reconstruction in the frontal axis, with detection of flows at different depths. Yet another advantage of OCTA over angiography is the ability to study different vascular planes at different depths. It will therefore enable us to assess not only the superficial vascular plexus (PVS), but also the middle (PVM) and deep (PVP)(4,5), making it possible to visualize the various chorio-retinal vascular structures, both normal and pathological, without the injection of contrast and in three dimensions. As a result, this non-invasive technique has further reduced the role of retinal dye angiography. Its applications have become increasingly numerous and will continue to grow.

2. ANALYSIS AND INTERPRETATION TECHNIQUES

2.1. Technical aspects :

The OCTA principle is based on the fact that "in a motionless eye, the only moving structures are the figurative elements of the blood". Thus, images are obtained thanks to the difference in contrast between the moving elements (blood elements) and the fixed elements (vascular walls) (5).

Blood flow is visualized by detecting changes in movement in a sequence of OCT scans using a super-luminescent diode (SLD). This technique is based on the principle of "speckel" interferometry using the decorrelation principle(1,4,6).

Figurative elements in the chorio-retinal blood are illuminated by a laser source. Light rays reflected in all directions with numerous interferences are used to acquire mainly :

- **Autocorrelation signal**: compares the signal with itself to detect the slightest change. Only identical signals are highlighted.
- **The decorrelation signal**: highlights different objects at different times corresponding to the flow inside the vessels.

In OCTA, a beam of light is scanned across a region of the eye. The amount of reflection is measured, and the analysis is then repeated one or more times. Pixel values recorded at two different time points are compared(5). Changes are attributed to the movement of erythrocytes in blood vessels.

Areas where blood flow is faster will show greater changes over a given period. But the exact relationship between this change and flow velocity depends on many parameters, such as the size of the OCT beam and the size of the blood vessel. OCTA technology is based on the detection of differences in amplitude, intensity or phase variance between sequential B-scans taken at the same point on the retina (7)(2).image acquisition is based on horizontal scans combined or not with vertical scans, depending on the device used. OCTA technologies have made it possible to divide the OCT spectrum into narrower bands, thus improving the signal-to-noise ratio, at the expense of axial resolution.

Thus, the OCTA image is different from that of structural OCT. It shows only the vessels in the vascularized retinal layers and in the choroid. In structural OCT, we speak of hypo- and hyperreflectivity, whereas in OCTA, the image is formed by a flow signal, so we speak of hyper or hypo flow signal(4,5).

Flux will be detectable above the threshold set by the device and will depend on the inter-scan interval. Most devices(2) detect flux within a fairly wide range, from 0.5 to 2 mm per second.

Several OCTA machines are available: the Cirrus 5000HD AngioPlexTM from Zeiss, the Optovue AngioVue from EBC Europe, the Heidelberg Spectralis OCTA from Sanotek(8), the OCTA triton from Topcon.

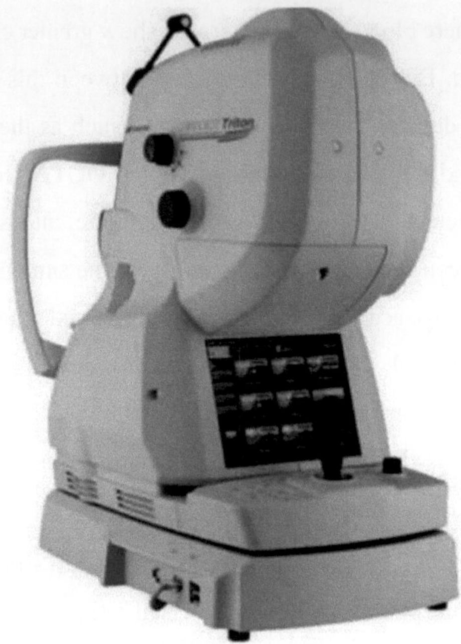

Figure 1: Triton OCT device from Topcon

The OCTA technique of this device is based on the principle of amplitude variation, using a source with a wavelength of 1050nm with an acquisition speed of 100,000 A scans/s, giving 320 horizontal scans for a 3*3 mm acquisition. The OCTA technique used is full spectrum swept sourceoptimized by OCT-A ratio analysis (OCTARA). This is a proprietary image-processing algorithm that provides high-sensitivity angiographic detection, with an eye-tracking system (smarttrack) that reduces artifacts during OCTA image acquisition(9). The device provides 8um axial resolution, 20um transverse resolution with axial digital resolution and 2.6um axial depth(4).

2.2. OCTA interpretation of normal fundus :

OCTA flow signals are acquired simultaneously with structural OCT, and flow analysis is performed in comparison with retinal structure in frontal and cross-sectional images. OCTA's ability to distinguish capillaries depends on image resolution. For SD-OCTA operating at 70 kHz/s, capillaries can be seen in a 6 × 6 mm cube, but resolution is optimal with a 3 × 3 mm cube. For SS-OCTA operating at 100 kHz/s, they can distinguish capillaries in 9 × 9 mm cubes, but mainly superficial capillaries (10).

OCTA interpretation requires a perfect understanding of the three-dimensional structure of the retinal capillary and choroidal vascular networks. To achieve this, the various layers must be clearly identified and segmented. This segmentation must be precise, and is fundamental to obtaining high-resolution images. It can be manual or automatic.

- ***Automatic segmentation***: there are algorithms which, by default, automatically segment the superficial retinal capillary network, the deep retinal capillary network, the outer retina and the chorio-capillary network. It's a rapid method that standardizes image capture. However, it is not without risk of segmentation error, especially in cases of architectural disorganization of the retinal and choroidal layers(6).
- ***Manual segmentation***: this is carried out using software incorporated into the devices. It enables automatic segmentation and its thickness to be modified, thus limiting layer intercalations

and providing a better analysis of the desired layer, particularly in the case of disorganized retinal and choroidal machine architecture(1,5,11).

2.2.1. Quality parameters

OCTA provides high-resolution images and enables us to assess the various chorio-retinal vascular networks: the superficial vascular plexus, the deep vascular plexus, the outer retina, the chorio-capillary and the choroid. The sensitivity of this new imaging technique also enables us to highlight the peripapillary capillaries located in the optic fibre layer, which has proved to be an interesting element in the diagnosis.

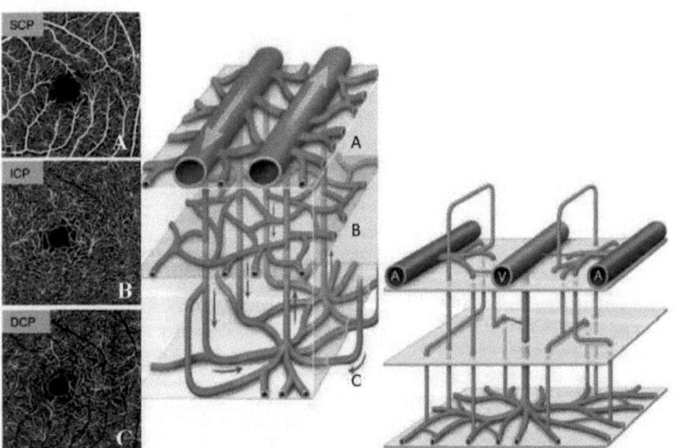

Figure 2: The different retinal vascular plexi between anatomical distribution and OCTA presentation: A :PVS/B :PVI/C :PVP

2.2.1.1. The PVS superficial vascular plexus (figure 3):

This plexus is located between the internal limiting membrane and the internal plexiform layer. This is the area visualized by 25um-thick C scan sections at the level of the ganglion cell layer(A).

The PVS is formed by the large vessels. The arteries (yellow arrows: B) are clearly identified, differing from the veins (green arrows: B) by the presence of a hypo-signal halo along their paths. PVS analysis revealed vessels with a continuous, linear shape and a homogeneous wall 75 um in diameter. This superficial network is characterized by its vascular density, with vessels evenly distributed like a spider's web, forming a 360° perifoveal vascular arcade that crowns the central avascular zone (ZAC) (red circle).

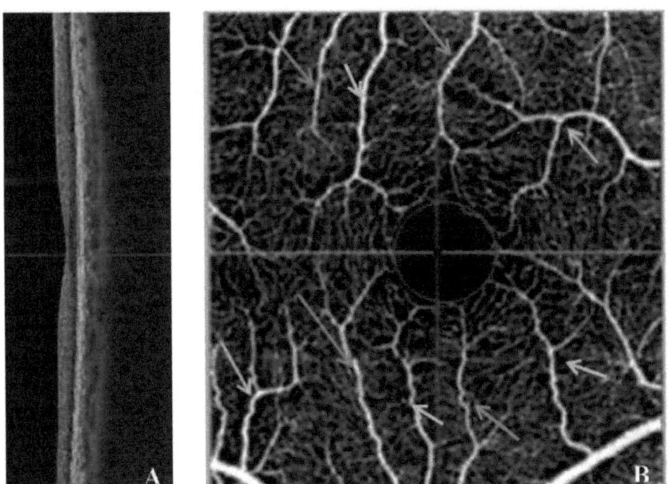

Figure 3: Appearance of normal PVS using 3*3 mm sections in a healthy subject

2.2.1.2. The PVI intermediate vascular plexus (figure 4):

Located between the superficial and deep plexus, below the internal limiting membrane. Thanks to OCTA, this plexus has become identifiable in vivo, in the form of a dense fine capillary network in the perifoveal region (6).

PVI capillaries form a three-dimensional network immersed in the thick inner plexiform layer. Their topography differs from that of superficial capillaries. In fact, there are no arterioles at this level, and the inner plexiform is crossed by venules originating from the outer plexiform, draining blood from the PVP, and to which the PVI capillaries connect.

This plexus has a regular distribution around the central avascular zone (CAZ): the anastomotic meshes are tighter and the interconnections are more complex, and the diameter of the CAZ is smaller than in the PVS. (1,7).

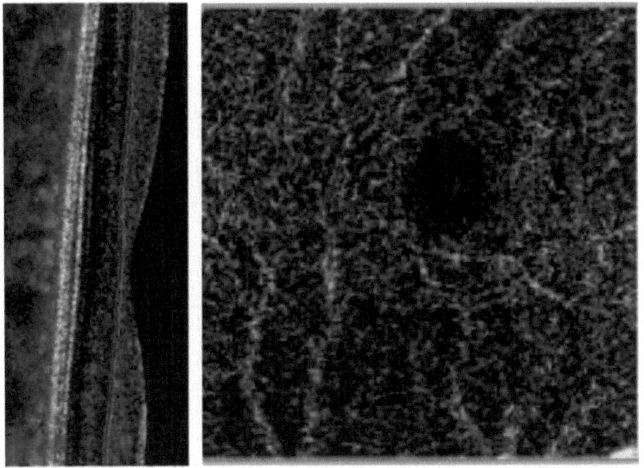

Figure 4: Normal PVI appearance using 3*3 mm sections in a healthy subject

2.2.1.3. The PVP deep vascular plexus (figure 5):

This vascular plexus is located between the inner and outer plexiform layers. The capillaries of the PVP are located in the outer plexiform layer. They are arranged in a single plane and organized in polygonal units that converge in a vortex towards a drainage venule that crosses the inner nuclear layer, the inner plexiform and the ganglion cell layer to drain into the superficial venules(2).

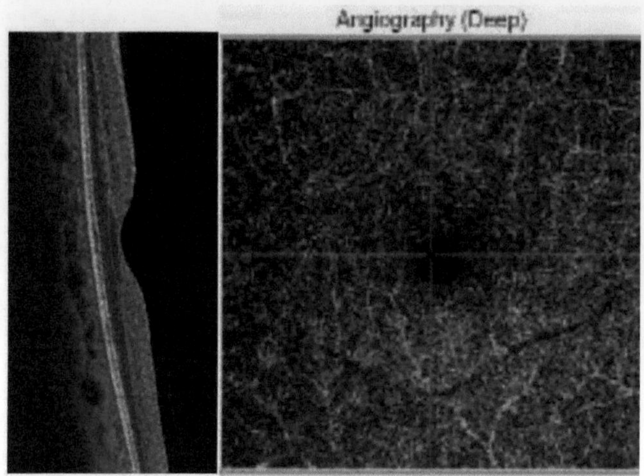

Figure 5: Normal appearance of the PVP in a healthy subject using 6*6mm sections

The ***deep*** vascular complex is formed by the intermediate and deep plexi. It is made up of relatively homogeneous capillaries, responsible for supplying the deep layers of the inner retina.

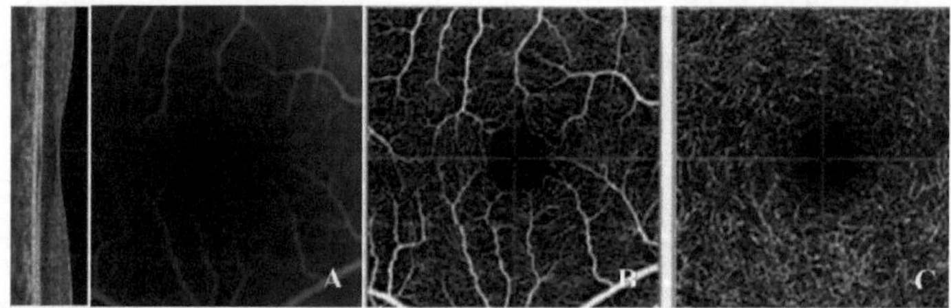

Figure 6: Comparison of different retinal vascular plexi in a normal subject in AF and OCTA using 3*3 mm sections. A: appearance in AF; B: PVS in OCTA; C: PVP in OCTA

We note the better individualization of vascular details in OCTA compared with FA, and the difference in capillary caliber and distribution. The ZAC appears narrower and tighter in the PVP than in the PVS and compared with FA.

2.2.1.4. The outer retina (figure 7):

Extends from the external plexiform to the pigment epithelium. It is normally avascular. There is an overlap of vascular functions between the 3plexi of the inner retina and the choroidal circulation to support the avascular outer retina, explaining its alternating hypo- and hyper-signal appearance.

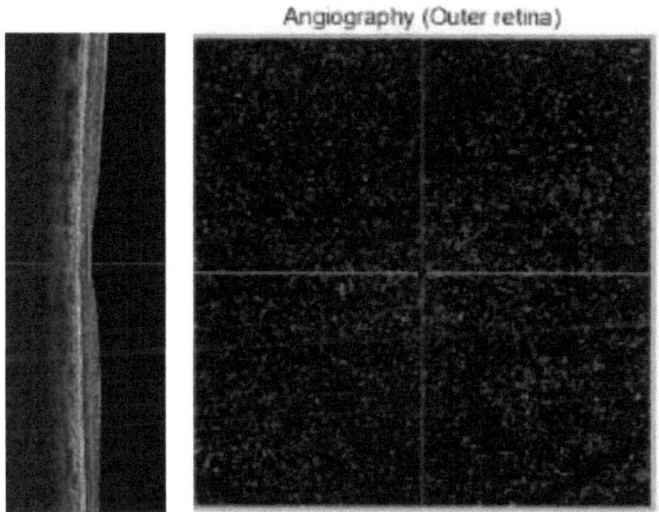

Figure 7: Normal appearance of the outer retina on OCTA (6*6mm) in a healthy subject

2.2.1.5. The chorio-capillary (figure 8):

It extends from Bruch's membrane to the 20um below. The OCTA shows a network of bright spots indicating the presence of a flow signal, and dark spots indicating the absence of flow. Interpretation of the normal chorio-capillary image remains difficult. On the one hand, the incident OCT signal is difracted by the pigment epithelium, and on the other, choroidal capillaries are relatively wide with very little inter-capillary space, making it difficult to detect their contours(2,7). However, this contrast between perfused and non-perfused areas becomes evident in cases of acute multi-focal choriocapillaris occlusion(12).

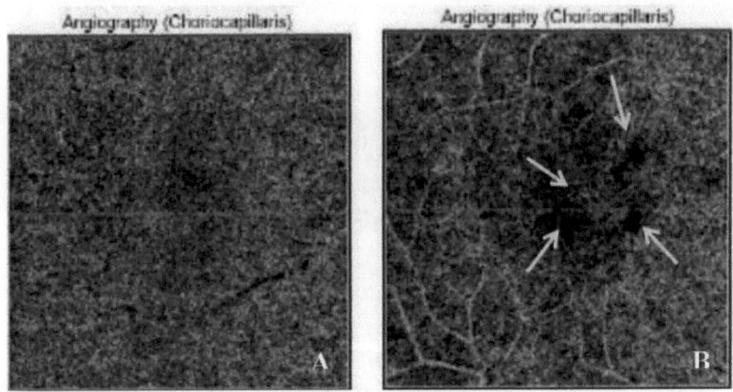

Figure 8: appearance of the Choriocapillaris in OCTA using slices (6*6mm)

A: normal 40-year-old subject B: 45-year-old subject with a history of poorly balanced hypertension complicated by hypertensive choroidopathy (areas of choroidal ischemia appearing as hypo flow signals (yellow arrows).

2.2.1.6. The choroid (figure 9/10):

In the normal eye, the large choroidal vessels are not visualized by OCTA. This is essentially due to the dispersion of the OCT light signal in the pigment epithelium and choriocapillaris (2,7).

- Sattler's layer: middle choroidal vascular layer. This capillary network is difficult to identify due to the attenuation of the signal from overlying structures.

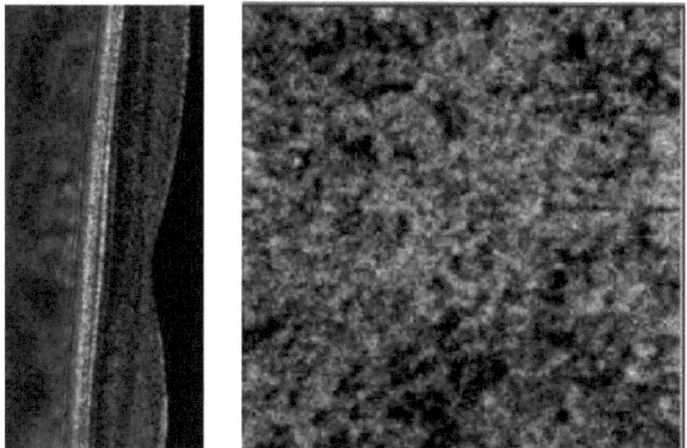

Figure 9: Manual segmentation of the Sattler layer in a normal subject using 3*3 mm sections

■ Haller's layer: appears as alternating zones of hypo and hyper signal, with a much wider vascular caliber than Sattler's layer.

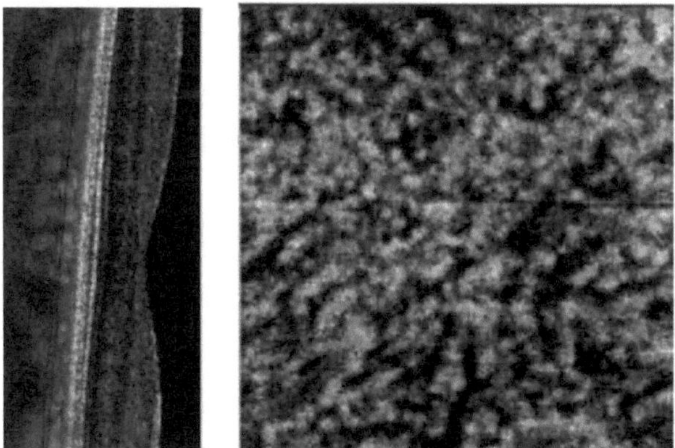

Figure 10: Manual segmentation of Haller's layer in a normal subject using 3*3 mm sections

2.2.2. Quantitative parameters

In addition to qualitative parameters, OCTA offers quantitative parameters for objective assessment of retinal abnormalities. These parameters provide new objective biomarkers, facilitating the diagnosis, monitoring and treatment of ocular pathologies(1,2,4,5).

- Vascular density(DV): is the percentage of surface area occupied by blood vessels. It differs according to the layer measured. Results can be expressed layer by layer for the entire 3 × 3 mm surface, or only for the ring-shaped para-foveal zone, or by quadrant of this zone(1,3).
- flow index(FI): is the average flow signal in the area studied. It provides an assessment of the vascular area in addition to blood flow velocity(2).
- The central avascular zone (CAZ): objective measurement of CAZ surface area and circularity index is a useful tool for assessing and monitoring diseases characterized by capillary loss, such as diabetic retinopathy(DR)(2,7).

2.3. OCTA artifacts:

Optimum detection of each capillary layer depends on accurate segmentation and the elimination of artifacts. Artifacts are more frequent with automatic segmentation, while manual segmentation minimizes acquisition and interpretation errors(13). Three main mechanisms are responsible for these artifacts: OCTA technology itself, data acquisition and image processing algorithms, and motion(9).

Various artifacts must be taken into account when interpreting images:

- **Projection artifacts**: these are fairly common and result from the combination of retinal vessel structure and OCT signal source(4,5,13). Mirror projection artefacts can arise from superficial retinal vessels, whose vessel lumen caliber fluctuates with the cardiac systolo-diastolic impulse. Another mechanism for projection artifacts is as follows: when incident light passes through the figurative elements of the moving blood (instead of being reflected), it passes through the blood vessels and reaches the underlying tissues. When this light reaches the EP, it is reflected and captured by the machine. The fraction of incident rays passing through the vessels varies over time, generating an artifactual decorrelation signal that is also responsible for projection artifacts(14). Vascular patterns in the superficial plexus are thus duplicated in the deep plexus, in the outer retina, which is normally avascular, or in the choriocapillaris(figure11). OCTA projection artifacts can lead to inaccurate measurement of the flow index and deeper retinal DV. In addition, they hamper the identification and quantification of NVCs in the outer retina, or may even be mistakenly recognized as NVCs. Software deletion of flow signals from projections leads to "negative" projections consisting of the same vascular pattern with a dark appearance of signal absence (4,13,14).

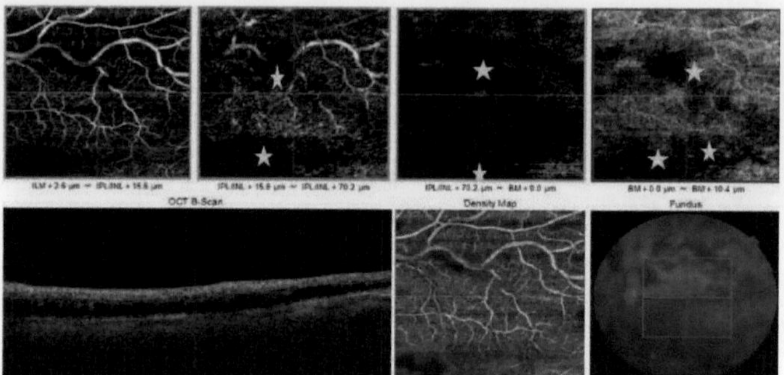

Figure 11: Projection artefact with artefact related to changes in the intrinsic properties of the eye :
Superficial vessels are duplicated in the deep plexus and choriocapillaris (red arrows).
Signal attenuation is noticeable in the PVP of the outer retina and in the choriocapillaris secondary to retinal hemorrhages (yellow stars).

- **Changes in the intrinsic properties of the eye** can generate artifacts either by masking or unmasking. In fact, dense ocular lesions such as haemorrhages, scars or pigments can attenuate or even block light, thus generating a weak signal (figure11). Retinal atrophy, on the other hand, is associated with increased reflectivity, enabling vessels to be seen more clearly through the unmasking effect(1,13,14).

- **Eye movement artifacts** :

Eye movements can produce white lines or a checkerboard pattern secondary to the juxtaposition of two different regions and different decorrelation indices. They can also produce images of stretched, doubled or spread vessels (figure12)(1,9,13). The use of eye-tracking is designed to limit fixation microartefacts and significantly improve decorrelation signal quality and contrast. However, its use slightly increases acquisition time, which may alter image quality(14).

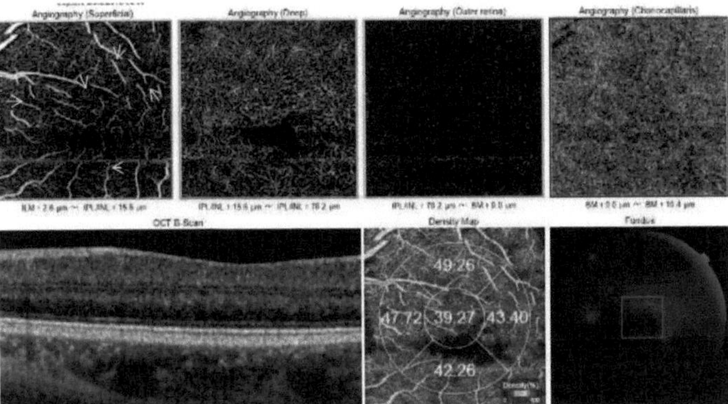

Figure 12: Motion artifact :
Image acquisition is not centered on the fovea. The vessels show a discontinuous path with forced alignment (yellow arrows).

➢ Segmentation artifacts

Since tiles are primarily defined by automatically segmented retinal layer boundaries, careful examination of segmentation is essential for correct interpretation. Segmentation failures are particularly common in diseases where the appearance and shape of the retinal layer is altered. For example, intra-retinal fluid, bulky PEDs, choroidal neovascularization and certain atrophies often cause segmentation errors. Manual correction facilitates and accelerates the correction of compromised slab boundaries using interactive segmentation correction processes(6,14-16).

3. OCTA AND DIABETIC RETINOPATHY

DR is the retinal localization of diabetic microangiopathy. It is a consequence of chronic hyperglycemia. Its first histological lesions are thickening of the basement membrane, loss of pericytes and then loss of endothelial cells in retinal capillaries, leading to their obstruction. In the vicinity of the small areas of capillary non-perfusion created, microaneurysms develop in the neighboring capillaries.

Dilatation and occlusion of retinal capillaries are the first clinically detectable lesions of DR, leading to two interrelated phenomena: hyperpermeability and occlusion, which evolve concomitantly. Hyperpermeability predominates in the central region, leading to macular edema, while occlusions mainly affect the peripheral retina, resulting in retinal ischemia. When retinal ischemia is extensive, neovessels proliferate, leading to neovascular complications such as preretinal hemorrhage, intravitreal hemorrhage, tractional retinal detachment, iritis rubeosis and neovascular glaucoma.

The diagnosis of DR is clinical, based on the bio-microscopic examination of the fundus. This enables us to identify the various signs of DR:

- microaneurysms and punctiform retinal haemorrhages are the first clinical signs of DR.
- cottony nodules indicate occlusion of the retinal precapillary arterioles.

- intra-retinal hemorrhages, venous anomalies such as irregular "rosary" venous dilatation or venous loops (omega veins) and intra-retinal microvascular anomalies (IRMA) are ophthalmoscopic signs suggestive of areas of non-perfusion and severe retinal ischemia.
- Pre-retinal and pre-papillary neovessels indicate proliferative DR.
- Retinal thickening in the macula indicates macular edema

When it comes to complementary examinations, FA remains the gold standard in DR. It provides a better assessment of these micro-vascular anomalies and a better quantification of retinal ischemia, thus helping in the classification and therapeutic management of DR (17-20). Nevertheless, the ability of FA to detect and analyze these capillary anomalies in detail is limited by the superposition of the different plexi and by the diffusion of the dye secondary to the often associated rupture of the blood-retinal barrier(21).

OCTA enables separate assessment of the superficial, intermediate and deep capillary plexi, unlike FA, which essentially maps the superficial retinal network. It can also explore the macular vascular network, particularly in the early stages of DR when FA is not indicated. All this makes OCTA an interesting technique for both the diagnosis and clinical investigation of DR(17).

3.1. OCTA and diabetic retinopathy

Clinical signs of DR can be analyzed using OCTA. OCTA provides high-definition images for precise analysis of microvascular alterations in diabetics.

3.1.1. Microaneurysms (figure 13)

They are visible on FO as punctiform red lesions with well-rounded borders, and on AF as focal dilatations of retinal capillaries. On B-scan OCT, the microaneurysm is visible in the inner retina (anatomical zone of retinal capillaries) as a rounded or oval lesion with sharp edges, classically hyporeflective content and typically with peripheral annular hyperreflectivity producing the ring sign(22).

On OCTA, microaneurysms appear as a rounded, saccular or fusiform decorrelation signal, measuring 14 to 136um in diameter, smaller than on FA due to the absence of dye diffusion and most often at the edge of a non-perfusion zone (20). They are more numerous in the deep bed than in the superficial plexus, confirming what has been demonstrated in histology and indicating that microvascular changes in diabetics are earlier and more severe in the PVP than in the PVS(17,23,24).However, the sensitivity of OCTA for detecting microaneurysms is lower than that of FA, and only 60% of microaneurysms visualized by FA are detected by OCTA(25). In fact, according to Viritti D et al(20), microaneurysms with hypo-reflective content on OCT B-scan appear to be detected less often on OCTA than those with moderate or hyper-reflective content. This suggests that either the blood flow in these lesions is too slow or turbulent and therefore unidentifiable, or that the aneurysm content is low in erythrocytes and/or partially thrombosed and this lack of flow is responsible for the absence of decorrelation signal, or because it is difficult to differentiate them from a vertical capillary section (22,25,26).

Given that microaneurysms are an early sign and important indicator of DR progression, the lack of detection of certain lesions could represent a drawback in the analysis of DR by OCTA (25).Interestingly, Hwang and collaborator showed that leaky areas at FA, attributed to large microaneurysms, were identified on OCTA as small clumps of protruding vertical neovascularization in the vitreous cavity(20,27).

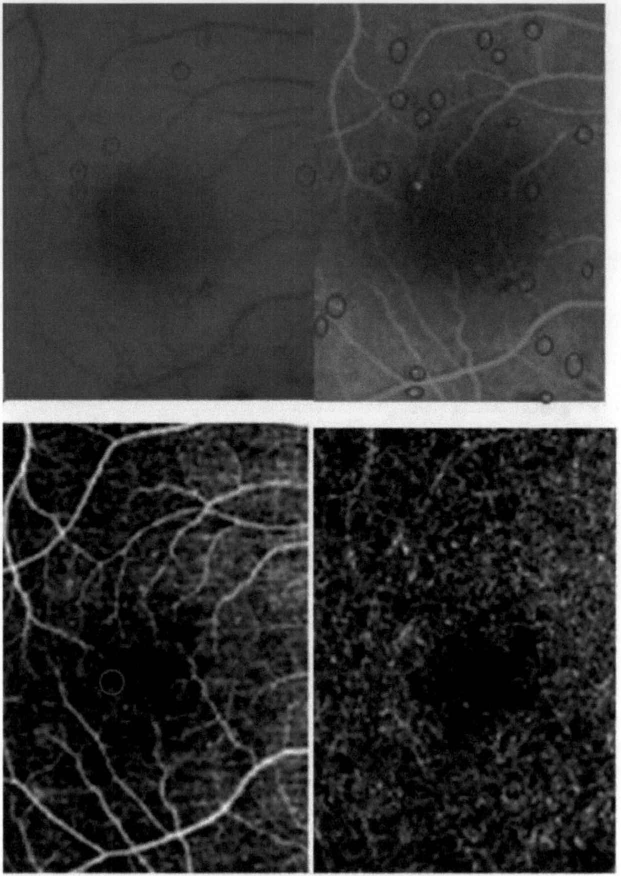

Figure 13: Microaneurysms between clinical appearance, AF and OCTA: 45-year-old with severe RDNP: microaneurysms (red circles) appear more numerous on AF than on clinical examination. On OCTA, microaneurysms in the PVS appear less numerous than in the PVP.

3.1.2. Microhemorrhages (figure 14):

On B-scan OCT, microhemorrhages appear as small, poorly defined, hyperreflective lesions in the inner layers of the retina (24).

In OCTA, since these are non-perfused lesions, they do not give a decorrelation signal, but may mask the capillary bed and give rise to a false appearance of focal rarefaction of flow(28).

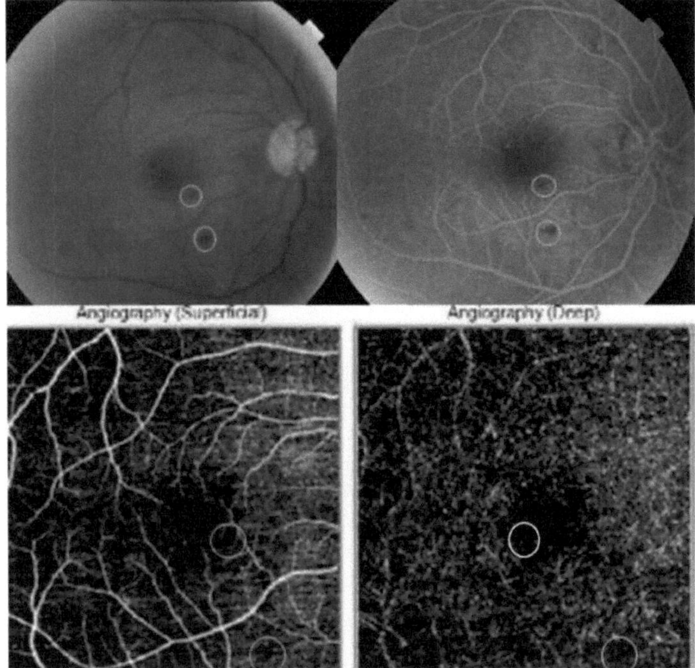

Figure 14: Translation of bleeding into FA and OCTA :
45 years old with non-proliferative DR: flaming haemorrhages in the peri-macular area (yellow circles) resulting in a masking effect in FA (hypo-fluorescent lesions) and in OCTA in a-signal lesions due to the absence of flux secondary to the masking of the decorrelation signal by the haemorrhages.

3.1.2. Cottony nodules :

They reflect occlusion of the retinal pre-capillary arterioles.

On B-scan OCT, the cottony nodules appear as a focal hyper-reflective nodular lesion of the inner retina, resulting in localized thickening of the optic fiber layer. On OCTA, no flow is detected within this hyper-reflective ischemic lesion(20).

3.1.3. Intraretinal microvascular anomalies (IRMAs) and preretinal and prepapillary neovessels (NVs):

AMIRs are vascular dilatations and telangiectasias developed in the periphery of territories of capillary occlusion; they would be intra-retinal neovessels. Pre-retinal and prepapillary neovessels appear as a vascular meshwork on the surface of the retina or papilla.

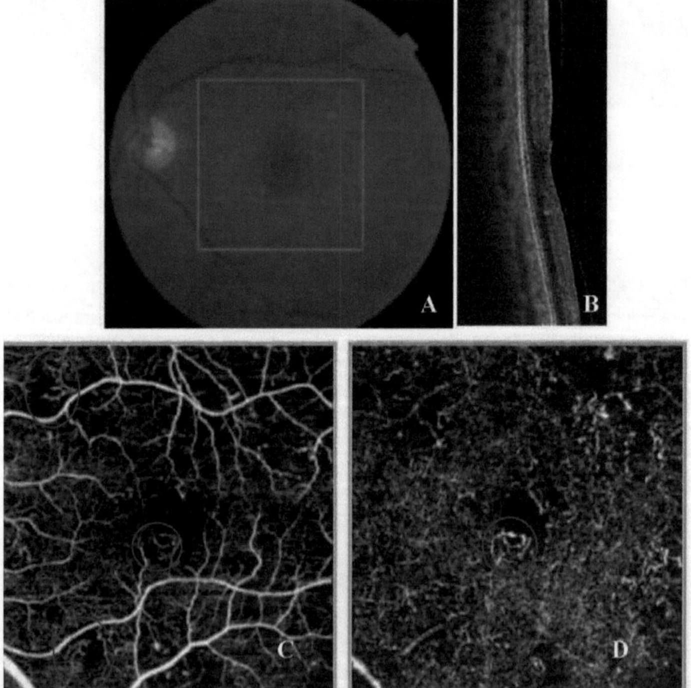

Figure 15: AMIRs visualized on the PVS and PVP :

Severe non-proliferative DR(A) with visualization of AMIR in the form of anarchic intraretinal vascular dilatations visualized at the PVS (C) and PVP(D) (red circles).

On OCT-B scan, neovessels are visible as hyperreflexia at the junction between the vitreous and the retina, unlike AMIR, which remain intraretinal(22,29).

In OCTA, these lesions are easily visible. This could be explained by the rapidity of blood circulation at their level on the one hand, and the absence of masking by dye diffusion on the other (30).

AMIR appear as abnormally dilated vessels in an extensive area of flow rarefaction, but remain in the retinal plane unlike neovessels. However, although they preferentially develop at the expense of the PVS, AMIR can also be visualized in the PVP layer, due to projection artifacts (31).

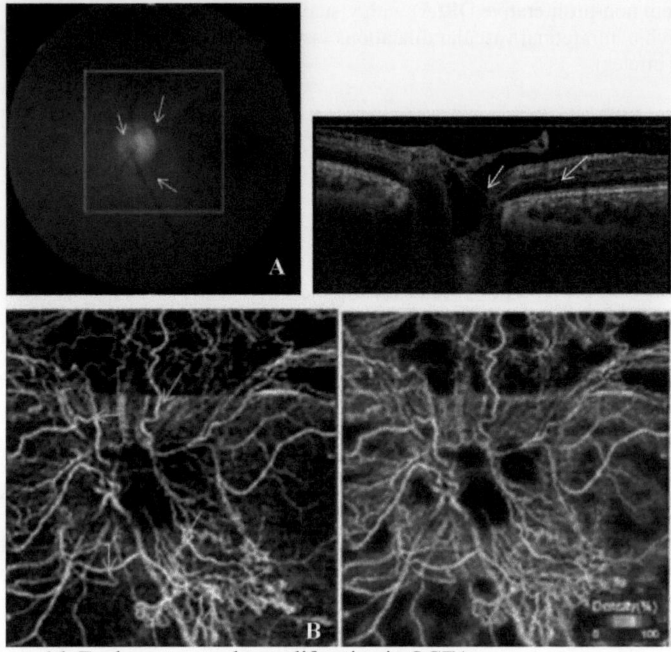

Figure 16: Exuberant vascular proliferation in OCTA :
Pre-papillary NV in a 47-year-old woman with treatment-naive ROP. Abnormal red blood columns can be seen on the optic nerve head (white arrows), but their detailed morphology is not clearly visible. (B): OCTA of the optic disc clearly shows the morphology of pre-papillary NV; vessels with large trunks (yellow arrows), terminal loops and anastomotic connections at the outer border of neovascularization (red stars). The most distinctive feature of this type of neovascularization is the exuberant vascular proliferation, which can be identified as an irregular proliferation of new small-caliber vessels.

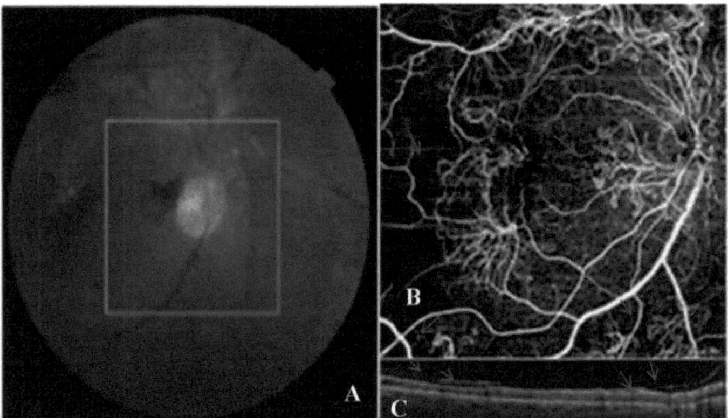

Figure 17: OCTA and RD FLORIDA : RD Florida in a 30-year-old female. A: the FO shows the presence of multiple fibrovascular proliferations occupying the entire posterior pole. (B) OCT section shows multiple vitreous hyperreflectivities associated with neovascular networks (red arrows). C: OCTA using 9*9 mm slices revealed accurate mapping of pre-retinal NV in the form of exuberant vascular proliferations (EVPs) (red arrows).

Another advantage of OCTA is that, with this technique, the edges of neovessels remain sharp due to the absence of dye diffusion, and the neovascular surface area can be quantified(32). As a result, this imaging technique can be used not only for diagnosis, but also as a non-invasive means of monitoring diabetic patients and assessing therapeutic efficacy. Indeed, Akihiro Ishibazawa and colleagues have shown that NVs in ROP patients can be morphologically divided into two main types: NVs with PVE and without PVE. EVP, which is the intense growth of small-calibre irregular vessels located at the margin of new vessels, probably represents active proliferation, as almost all treatment-naive eyes with RDP (95%) had lesions with EVP. This rate decreases steadily over the course of treatment(33).

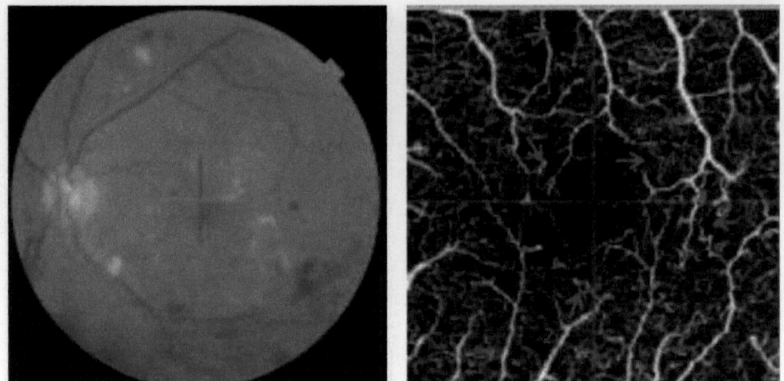

Figure 18: The different elementary lesions of diabetes in OCTA :
1 micro aneurysm
2 vascular loop
3 : AMIR
4 : breaking off the ZAC
5 zone of ischemia

OCTA therefore appears to be an interesting imaging tool for diabetic patients. However, the field of view is virtually the only real limitation of this technique in DR. Nevertheless, current A-OCT systems allow automatic combination and reconstruction of the acquired images, enabling good visualization of the posterior retina and middle periphery (26).

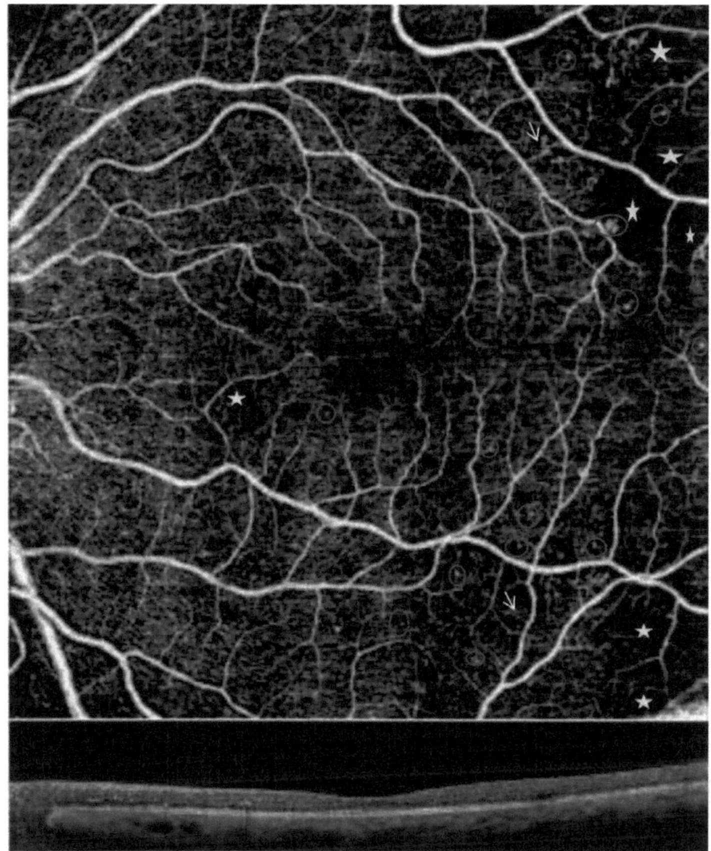

Figure 19: Overview of the PVS of a diabetic patient using 9*9 mm sections when fluorescein injection is contraindicated: Microaneurysms (red circles), areas of ischemia (yellow stars). AMIR (white arrows)

3.2. Diabetic macular edema

This is the accumulation of extracellular fluid in the macular retina, leading to its thickening. Thickening is associated, to varying degrees, with other lesions, principally intra-retinal logetes, but also retinal serous detachment (RSD), exudates, capillary occlusions and abnormalities of the vitreo-macular interface.

Given the early and sometimes intense diffusion present in AF, OCTA therefore appears to be the examination of choice for studying the vascular changes associated with DME.

3.2.1. Contribution of OCTA in the pathogenesis of diabetic macular edema :

Under normal conditions, excess fluids are eliminated to the vitreous cavity or to the PVS or PVP via aqueous (aquaporins) and potassium channels. In the case of DME, the internal blood-retinal barrier is disrupted and fluid diffuses into the retinal tissue.

According to Spaide et all (34), due to the probably lower hydrostatic pressure in the PVP, there would be a flow of fluid from the PVS to the PVP, where it would be reabsorbed, if the latter is intact. In the event of capillary occlusion in the PVP, reabsorption mechanisms would be impaired and fluid would accumulate in the form of intraretinal cysts in areas of deep capillary occlusion (figure 20).

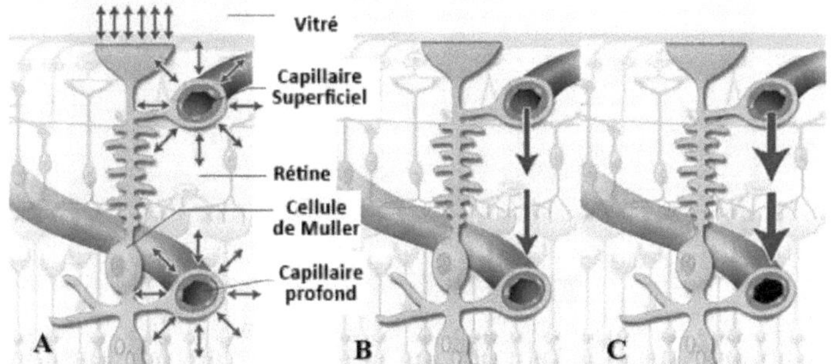

Figure 20: Pathogenesis of retinal edema: A: Under normal conditions. B**:** In the event of rupture of the inner blood-retinal barrier **C:** In the event of occlusion of deep plexus capillaries

3.2.2. Exudates (figure 21/22):

These are lipid accumulations within the retina. They are yellow deposits, arranged in a ring around microvascular anomalies (microaneurysms or (AMIR)).

On B-scan OCT, exudates are located mainly in the outer nuclear and plexiform layers and are highly hyper-reflective, with sharp edges and a marked shadow cone (figure 21). On OCTA, they appear paradoxically hyper-signal due to reflection of the decorrelation signal from perfused vessels located anteriorly (figure 22).

These exudates, especially small ones, can be mistaken for microaneurysms. Simultaneous analysis of OCT-B scan and OCTA can help distinguish between the two(20).

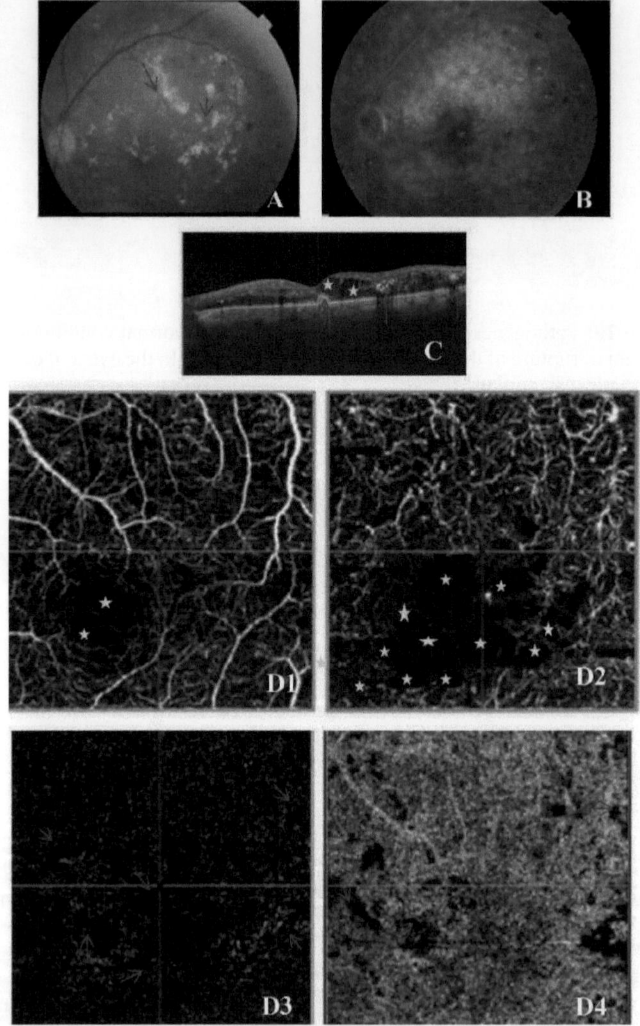

Figure 21: Deep exudates in OCTA.

A 70-year-old woman: FO: severe RDNP with clinically significant macular edema and deep exudative plaques (red arrows) (A).AF: deep exudates with no angiographic translation (B). OCT SD: diffuse retinal thickening with hyporeflective edema pockets (yellow stars) and hyperreflective deep exudates with posterior shading (red arrows) (C).

OCTA: exudates are untranslated in the PVS (D1) and PVP (D2); in the outer retina (D3), exudates mask the decorrelation signal (red arrows). Choriocapillaris (D4): overall rarefaction of the vascularization, with areas of hypo signal secondary to masking due to the presence of cystoid logettes and a signal secondary to deep exudates.

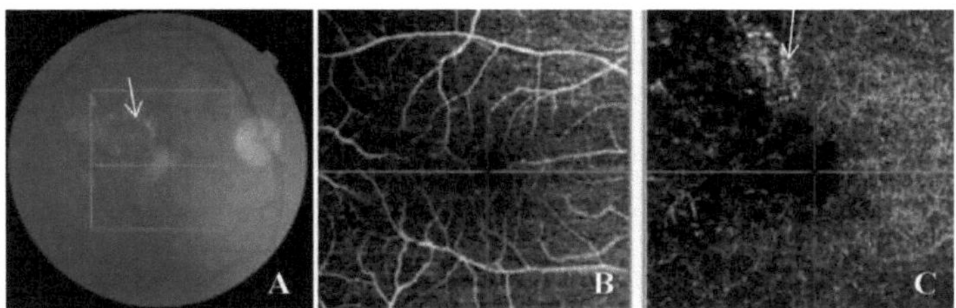

Figure 22: Lipid exudates and artifactual decorrelation hyper signal.
Lipid exudates (A) were not translated at the PVS level of the OCTA with an artefactual hyper signal at the PVP level (C) (white arrows).

3.2.4: Macular edema logettes (figure 23)

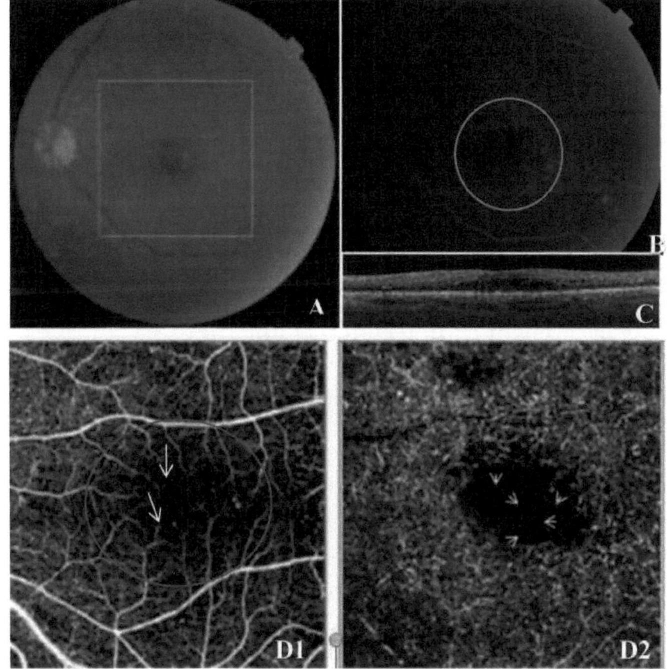

Figure 23: OCTA and cystoid logettes
Moderate non-proliferative RD with cystoid OM (A). The cystoid logettes are

seen in FA as honeycomb-shaped impregnation of the logettes(B), in OCT B scan as round hypo-reflexia of different sizes, in OCTA as widening of the ZAC with rupture of the perifoveal anastomotic circle at the level of the PVS (white arrow)(D1).The cystoid logettes are best evidenced at the level of the PVP as a-signal areas on a background of hypo-perfusion in hypo-perfusion.

signal (blue circles) separated by hypo-signal traverses (yellow arrows) secondary to areas repressed by cystoid logettes(D2).

These are intra-retinal cystic lesions linked to the accumulation of fluid in the retinal extracellular compartment, and are associated with microaneurysms and widening of the ZAC.

On B-scan OCT, the logettes are rounded or ovoid, variable in size and hyporeflective in content (35)(figure 21/23). On OCTA, logettes are also rounded or oval, black, totally devoid of flow signal, located close to territories of microvascular anomalies and associated with decreased capillary density in both deep and superficial plexi. They are more frequent and more extensive in the PVP, and are perfectly superimposed on the logettes present on the OCT B-scan.

After cure of DME, areas previously occupied by cysts remain devoid of capillaries, and logetes will preferentially reappear in these areas in the event of DME recurrence(36).

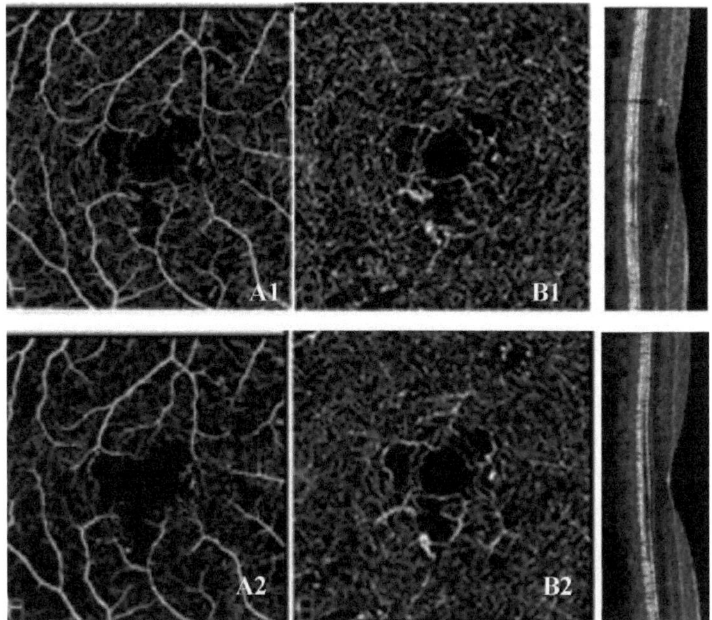

Figure 24: Appearance of the various retinal vascular plexi after treatment with anti VEGF (37) :

A1/B1: OCT B scan slices through the PVS (A1: before anti VEGF treatment.B1: after anti VEGF treatment.

A2/B2: PVP A2 before treatment. B2 after treatment.

A3/B3: PVP A3 before treatment. B3 after treatment.

On B scans, the cystoid logettes disappeared, along with the OMD. OCTA slices show the presence of an enlarged ZAC after treatment, with a rupture of the perifoveal anastomotic circle (yellow arrows) that predominates at the PVS level, with a decrease in DV (perimacular capillary loss) (red circles).

3.3. Quantification of the central avascular zone

Thanks to OCTA, it is also possible to visualize areas of macular capillary non-perfusion more precisely, and to obtain values and a map of this density.

In DR, mean macular capillary density is lowered in both superficial and deep plexi. This density is correlated with the severity of DR (35)(38). As a result, the evolution of DR can be monitored by measuring the evolution of the ZAC, and any progressive widening of the ZAC is a sign of the severity of DR (39).

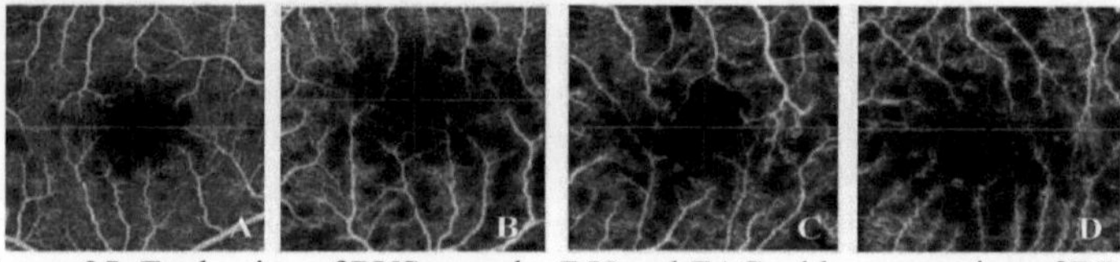

Figure 25: Evaluation of PVS macular DV and ZAC with progression of DR in subjects of the same age.
A: diabetic subject with no sign of DR, B: subject with moderate DR, C: subject with severe DR, D: subject with ROP. We note the decrease in vascular density in the PVS with the progression of DR, with widening of the ZAC and rupture of the perifoveal anastomotic circle.

Furthermore, an anatomical-functional correlation between capillary density and visual acuity (VA) has been demonstrated. Indeed, Samara et al (40) reported a negative correlation between VA and vascular density in the PVS and PVP, while Dupas et all (41) suggested that this correlation is essentially with the PVP.

3.4. Alterations to the capillary bed (Figure 25 -26) :

With OCTA, confocal analysis of the different vascular planes is possible. As a result, early changes in the capillary bed of the PVS, PVI and PVP could be identified even in the sub-clinical stages of DR.

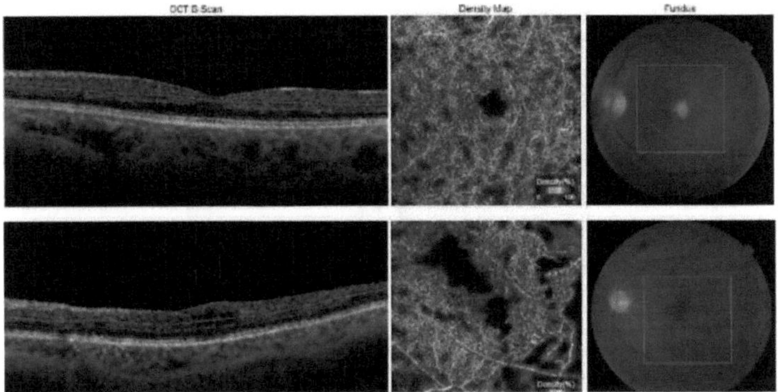

Figure 26: Comparison of PVP vascular density between a diabetic patient with no signs of DR and a diabetic patient with severe non-proliferative DR.

We note the decrease in vascular density in the PVP, with areas of no flow in blue contrasting with areas of hyperflow all around.

In DR, all plexi are affected. However, capillary involvement in PVP is always earlier and more severe than in PVS(23,25). On the other hand, micro-vascular involvement is specific to each plexus:

- **In the superficial plexus**, there is capillary rarefaction with areas of non-perfusion, appearing as irregular grey areas bounded longitudinally by capillaries (42). And, as already demonstrated, the ZAC is enlarged compared with normal subjects.

- **In the deep plexus**, capillary density is lowered overall, but with areas of non-perfusion that are less well defined. Moreover, the normal vortex architecture described by Bonnin et al (43) is no longer respected, and disorganization of the PVP is systematically found.

3.5: CHOROIDAL ANOMALIES

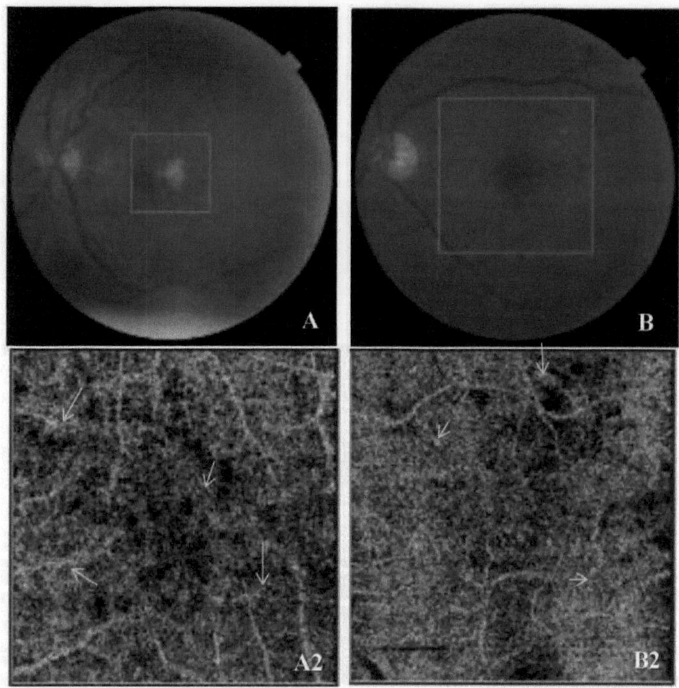

Figure 27: OCTA and vascular changes of the Choriocapillaris during DR. Al: moderate non-proliferative RD in a 52-year-old patient.B1: 3*3 mm OCTA section of the coriocapillaris. A2: pre-proliferative DR in a 45-year-old patient. B2: 6*6 mm OCTA section of the choriocapillaris.
We note the presence of a decrease in DV with areas of ischemia in hyposignal (yellow arrows) with choriocapillary vascular dilatations (red arrows).

Choroidal changes in diabetic patients have been

demonstrated(44,45) and OCT has enabled these choroidal changes to be assessed non-invasively and quantitatively.

On OCT-B scan, choroidal thinning, particularly of the choriocapillaris and the retrofoveolar medium vessel layer, was observed (46).

For OCTA, choroidal analysis is better with SS-OCTA(47). Indeed, with SD-OCTA, it is limited by the hyperreflectivity of the pigment epithelium and the hyper signal of the choriocapillaris. This analysis showed the presence of vascular remodeling with irregular, tortuous choroidal vessels close to histological descriptions(48)and a decrease in the vascular density of the choriocapillaris(figure 27)(49,50). Choroidal vascular density and volume are inversely correlated with the degree of severity of DR (47).

3.6. Contribution of OCTA in the absence of clinical signs of DR (figure28-29):

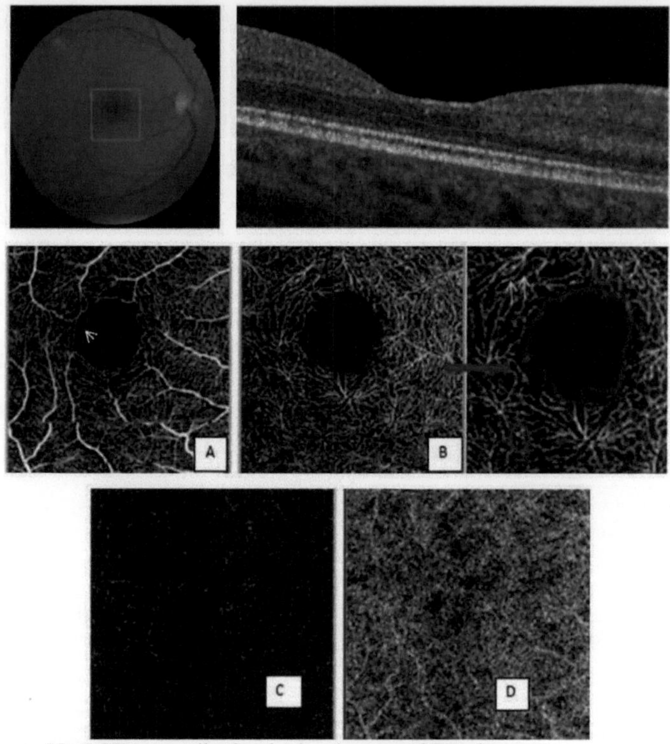

Figure 28: OCTA contribution in the absence of DR signs
The patient was 55 years old and had been diabetic for 7 years, with no signs of DR on the FO. OCTA: 3*3 mm slice: a zone of rupture of the perifoveal anastomotic circle is seen in the PVS. In the PVP, vascular dilatation (yellow arrows) with enlargement of the ZAC, which appears larger than its size in the PVS (B), and areas of hypointensity hypoperfusion in the choriocapillaris (red arrows) (D).

OCTA enables capillary alterations to be detected even before signs of DR appear on clinical examination and FA(7). This technique has revealed abnormalities that predominate in the PVP but also affect the PVS and Choriocapillaris, confirming the pathophysiological findings on histopathological sections (8). OCTA revealed a decrease in capillary density, visualization of microaneurysms with capillary rarefaction at their level, and irregularity of the FAZ with or without an increase in diameter(8,22). This could make it a possible means of screening for diabetic retinopathy before the appearance of the slightest clinical sign (39).

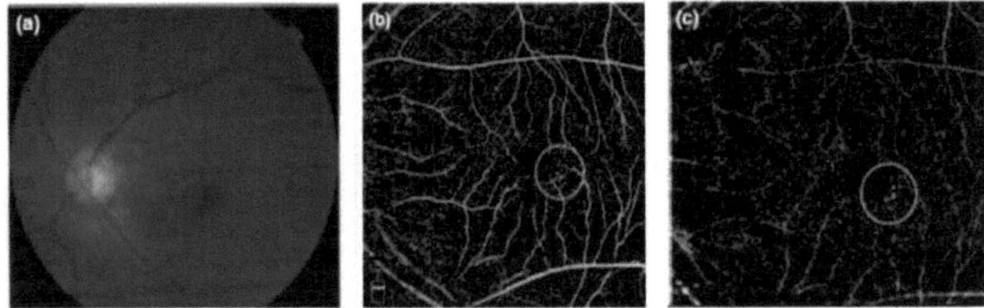

Figure 29: OCTA microaneurysms in the absence of DR signs
Typical case of a patient with no signs of DR on the FO who presents microaneurysms (yellow circles) that are objectivable by OCTA in the PVS and PVP (40).

4. OCTA AND AGE-RELATED MACULAR DEGENERATION

Age-related macular degeneration (AMD) is a group of degenerative, non-inflammatory, acquired lesions of the macular region occurring in a previously normal eye in subjects over the age of 50, and resulting in macular changes variously associating abnormalities of the EP and sensory retina and/or drusen and NVC (51). It is a serious and blinding pathology, representing the leading cause of visual impairment after the age of 50 in industrialized countries.

Pathophysiologically, AMD is of unknown etiology. Its main risk factors, apart from age, are hereditary factors and smoking. Dysfunction of the functional unit: EP - Mb de Bruch - choriocapillaris constitutes its primum movens (52).

This is a progressive disease, with early stages grouped under the term age-related maculopathy (AMD), with no functional repercussions, and late stages with impairment of central visual function, in which two forms are distinguished: exudative and atrophic AMD. It is possible to go from an exudative form to an atrophic one, and vice versa, or even for both to coexist.

4.1. OCTA and age-related maculopathy:

MLA is the early form of AMD. Although it can remain stable and does not systematically evolve into AMD, its existence is a risk factor and warrants careful monitoring.

MLA is clinically characterized by PE alterations and drusen. PE changes may be hyperpigmented or hypopigmented, and drusen may be miliary, serous isolated or confluent, pseudodrusen reticulated, cuticular, retractile or ghost drusen(53).

Previously, MLA monitoring was based on color fundus photographs. With the advent of OCT, the latter has become the reference examination for drusen analysis.

In OCTA, drusen in most cases give rise to artifacts and a masking effect of the choriocapillaris. However, this imaging technique can provide information on choriocapillaris perfusion and the neovascular risk of lesions(53,54).

> **Serous drusen (figure 30)**:

They are frequent, bulky, irregular in shape and blurred in outline.

On OCT-B scan, they appear as multiple domed elevations of the EP, moderately reflective. They may merge to form the drusenoid detachment of the PE, in the form of a bumpy, irregular uplift with hyper-reflective content.

In OCTA, these drusen most often lead to attenuation of the choriocapillaris signal and segmentation errors (55).

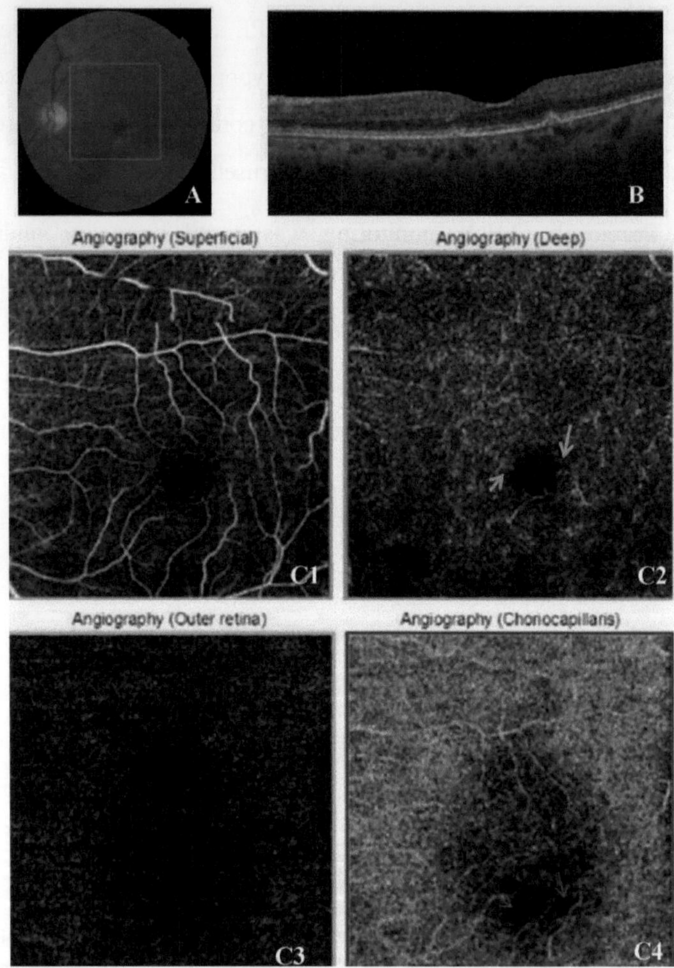

Figure 30: OCTA and serous drusen.

The FO of a 65-year-old female patient shows peri-macular confluent serous drusen(A). OCTB scan shows hyperreflective elevations of the EP in relation to the drusen(B) .OCTA shows a normal appearance of the PVS(C1). In the PVP, the perifoveal anastomotic circle is broken (green arrows), with widening of the ZAC. There are also abnormal vascular dilatations in the peri-macular area (red circles)(C2). In the choriocapillaris, drusen appear as a-signal areas in a hypo-signal range, related to a decrease in the vascular density of the choriocapillaris that exceeds the limits of the drusen (red circle).drusen appear as a-signal areas (red arrows) due to attenuation of the choriocapillaris signal.

- **Pseudo-drusen reticules or blue drusen (figure 31):**

They are yellowish, preferentially located in the upper temporal arches.

On OCT B scan, they are dense, hyper-reflective, located anterior to the EP and associated with a thinned choroid (56).

With OCTA, a considerable decrease in vascular density and decorrelation signal index at the level of the choriocapillaris associated with larger areas of non-perfusion have been demonstrated (55,57).

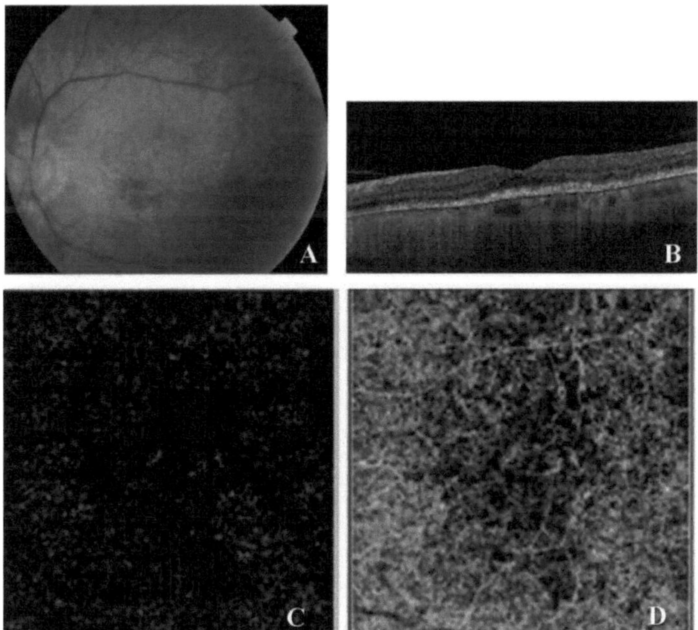

Figure 31: OCTA and reticulated pseudo drusen

This is a 62-year-old woman who presented with progressive BAV in both eyes. Examination of the FO revealed small, yellowish drusen occupying the entire posterior pole in favor of drusenreticularis (A).
The OCT B scan shows the presence of hyper-reflective irregularities in the EP(B). The OCTA shows, in the choriocapillaris (D), areas of hypo perfusion in hypo signal with signal masking secondary to the presence of drusen. There are also abnormal hyper-signal vascular dilatations of the choriocapillaris between the drusen (red arrows).

➢ **Vascularized drusen (figure 32/33)**:

This is an entity recently described with OCTA. These lesions mimic serous drusen, but are associated with a hyper-signal of the choriocapillaris. At first, they were considered to be type 1 macular neovascularization, but later they were found with intermediate AMD, raising the problem of differential diagnosis between large drusen and slowly progressive type 1 neovascularization(55,58,59).

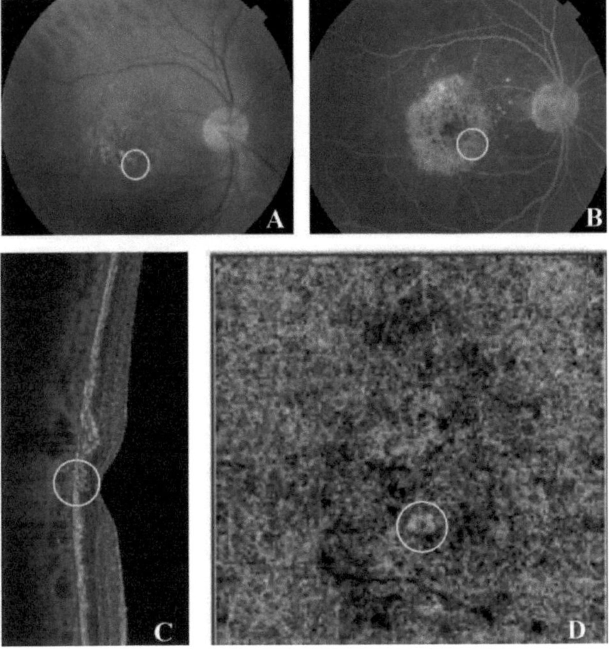

Figure 32: Vascularized drusen on multimodal imaging1.

A large yellowish drusenoid lesion (red arrow) with confluent small drusenoid lesions (yellow circle) is visible on FO(A). On the FA, we note the presence of macular hyper-fluorescence due to the window effect, with hypo-fluorescent lesions corresponding to drusen without hyper-fluorescence secondary to NVC (B). OCT sections show a dome-shaped drusenoid EPD with heterogeneous EP hyper-reflectivity corresponding to confluent drusen (C). OCTA of the choriocapillaris shows a neovascular hyper-signal network, corresponding to the flow signal within the confluent drusen(D).

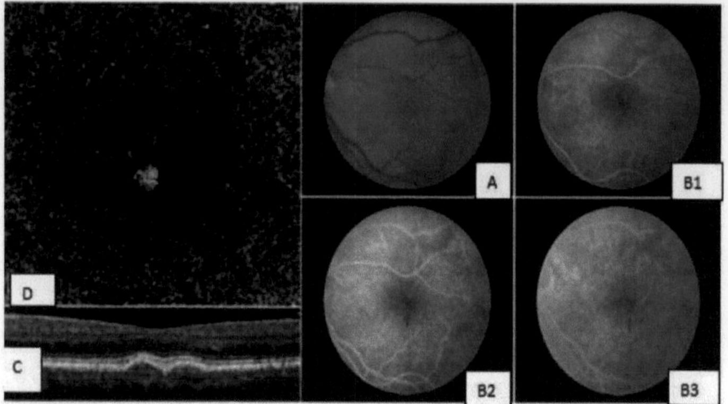

Figure 33: Vascularized drusen on multimodal imaging 2 (60).
A typical yellow drusenoid lesion is noted on the FO image (red arrows). On FA, no obvious hyper-fluorescence (red arrows B1/B2/B3). OCT(C) shows dome-shaped drusenoid EP elevation with heterogeneous multi-laminar sub-EP hyper-reflectivity. OCTA (D) shows a neovascular network, corresponding to the outflow signal located within the drusenoid lesion. Manual segmentation of the EP and Bruch's membrane was used to clearly visualize the neovascular network.

Thus, drusen are associated with a reduction in choriocapillary blood flow, which takes on a mottled appearance with alternating areas of hypo- and hyper-signal. This hypo-perfusion is associated with a widening of the ZAC with capillary rarefaction and rupture of the perifoveal anastomotic circle(61). These alterations are essentially age-related(62), but the presence of drusen seems to aggravate the extent of hypo-perfusion zones.

The reduction in vascular density is proportional to the extent of the drusen, their size, arrangement and, above all, their confluence, and areas of hypo-perfusion may extend beyond the boundaries of the drusen. Vascular density is also proportional to alterations in ellipsoid zones, which are essential areas of drusen focus(63).

4.2. Atrophic age-related macular degeneration (figure34):

This is a chronic pathology characterized by the progressive disappearance of retinal cells, particularly photoreceptors, and sometimes the entire macular retinal tissue. Diagnosis is clinical, with localized retinal discoloration and abnormal visualization of choroidal vessels.

Histologically, atrophic AMD is characterized by the loss of the EP, the outer layers of the neurosensory retina and the choriocapillaris in the macula.

OCT-B scan provides quantitative and qualitative evidence of these structural abnormalities. It shows hyper-reflectivity of the choroidal layers in atrophic areas. This hyper-reflectivity is due to the accentuated visualization of the choroid secondary to the disappearance of the PE. This phenomenon seems to be enhanced by retinal thinning, sometimes associated with atrophic areas of choriocapillaris and PE(53).

In atrophic AMD, OCTA shows hypo-perfusion in the superficial and deep vascular plexuses, associated with rarefaction or even disappearance of the choriocapillaris, consistent with the anomalies reported by OCT-B scan. It can also be used to delineate areas of geographic atrophy(52,63,64). This enables OCTA to correlate vascular changes with structural changes and monitor them in vivo. However, this fine tomographic analysis must be combined with multimodal imaging to better anticipate the rate of progression of this AMD and avoid misinterpretation and projection artifacts.

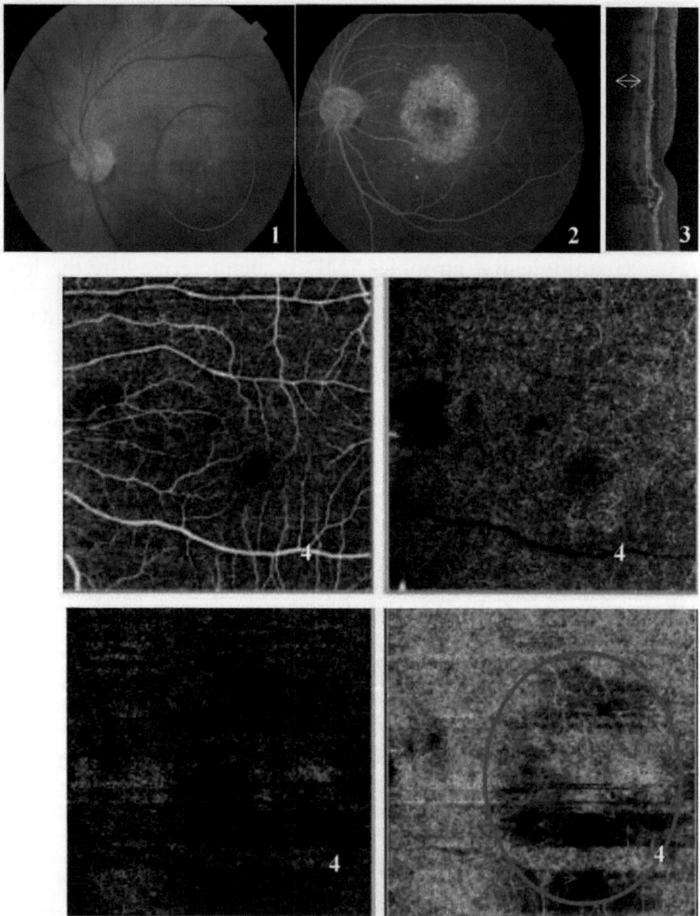

Figure 34: OCTA AND atrophic AMD.
65-year-old man followed for trophic AMD: FO (1): multiple serous drusen on a background of retinal atrophy. The FA showed the limits of this atrophic zone, with the presence of peripheral drusen and alterations in the EP beyond the

atrophic zone(2). On SD OCT, choroidal atrophy with drusenoidal EPDs(3). On OCTA, the architecture of the PVS is preserved (4a), with the presence of abnormal vascular dilatations in the PVP (4b).in the choriocapillaris, there is a hypo-signal area secondary to choriocapillaris atrophy, with abnormal visibility of the choroidal vessels.

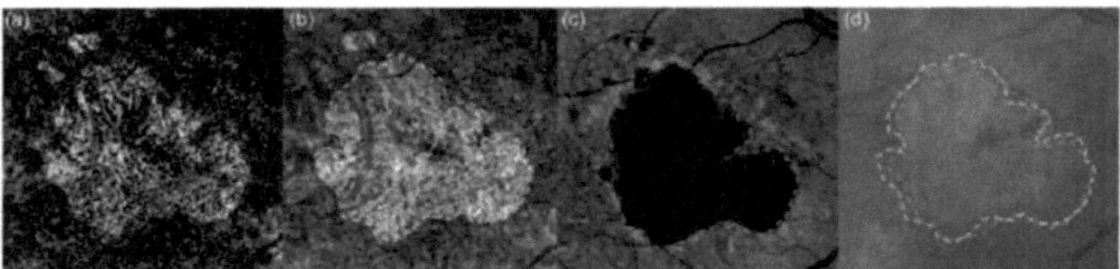

Figure 35: Comparison of imaging modalities for the delineation of geographic atrophy lesions(65)
(a) OCTA of the choriocapillaris. (b) SD-OCT of the choriocapillaris. (c) FO autofluorescence. (d)Comparison of geographic atrophy zone delineations for different modalities superimposed on the corresponding color FO photograph.

4.3. Exudative AMD

It is characterized by the abnormal proliferation of small blood vessels in the macular region. These "neovessels" are either choroidal or deep retinal in origin, and proliferate into the sub-retinal space or under the EP(66).

Neovessels are immature, with permeable walls. This leads to the accumulation of serous fluid and/or haemorrhage between the EP and the neuroretina, causing DSR, and/or between the EP and the MB, causing DEP. On the other hand, this neovascular proliferation may lead to alterations and remodelling of the retinal extracellular spaces, resulting in intraretinal edema (67).

FA is the gold standard for the investigation of exudative AMD (49,50). However, dye impregnation and diffusion can generate images that are difficult to interpret.

The advent of structural OCT represented a revolution in AMD imaging and is now widely used in the exploration and follow-up of neovascular AMD. It allows precise visualization of abnormalities, specifying their topography and quantifying them(51,68,69).

However, clear differentiation between hyper-reflective neovascular or fibrous structures is sometimes difficult. On the other hand, OCT, like FA, only allows indirect visualization of the neovessel through the presence of intra- or subretinal fluid, but the precise location and morphology of the CVN is difficult to assess (54).

For the first time, OCTA enables precise morphological analysis of CVNs. What's more, thanks to its ability to visualize vascular pathways, neovessels of choroidal origin that progressively develop in front of or under the PE can be detected very early with OCTA.

4.3.1. Neovessel appearance in OCTA :

OCTA will show a high, abnormal neovascular "flow" in a known vascular architecture.

The description of the main aspects of neovessels is based on neovessel activity criteria(70). The activity criteria for neovessels in OCTA are divided into 5 criteria:

> The shape

> Branching pattern

> Anastomoses and loops

> Vessel termini

> Peri-lesional hypo-intense halo: considered as a region of choriocapillaris alteration or flow impairment and/or localized atrophy.

We can thus distinguish between "active" forms requiring treatment, "quiescent" forms requiring monitoring, and inactive forms:

- **Active NV**: fine, tortuous, tangled, dense, interconnected capillaries with loops and anastomoses, connected by a peripheral neovascular anastomotic arch, anterior to Bruch's membrane. This network is surrounded by a dark peri-lesional halo at the level of the segmentation on Bruch's membrane.
- **Inactive NV**: mature, sparsely-dense, linear, voluminous, rarefied vessels, centrifugally arranged, without fine branches or peripheral arch.
- **Quiescent NV**: without functional and/or exudative manifestations (figure 36)

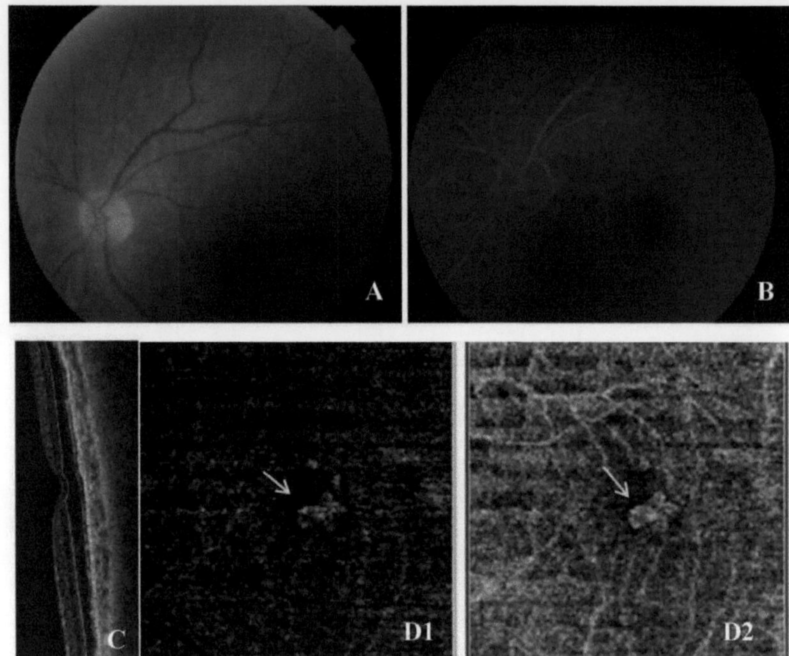

Figure 36: OCTA appearance of quiescent NVC.
68-year-old patient with stable AMD, no exudative signs on FO(A), no hyper fluorescence with diffusion on FA(B). OCT B scans showed no evidence of choroidal neo-vessels(C). OCTA revealed a small, hyper-reflective neovascular lacis with no visible capillary detail, and no peripheral peri-lesional halo: this is more likely to be a quiescent neo-vessel (D1/D2).

Table I: Criteria for neovessel activity in OCTA(69-74)

	NV active	NV inactive	NV quiescent
Shape	Well-defined, tortuous, wheel-shaped or sea-fan-shaped	As a "dead tree	Well-defined with a *core* and a peripheral ring *(margin)* Linear NV (long and filamentous)
Tree	numerous fine capillaries	Rare, voluminous, linear vessels, Centrifugal	Fine interconnected branches
Anastomoses and loops	Present	Absent	Often present
Peripheral anastomotic arch	Present	Absent	often present or partial
Somber perilesional halo	Often present	Absent	Often present
Flux localization on colorized OCT B-scan	High flow ahead of Bruch	Flow ahead of the Bruch	Low flow in front of the Bruch, high, localized choroidal flow

OCTA has its place in the initial assessment of exudative AMD. It provides qualitative and quantitative information with high sensitivity and specificity(70,75-77). Indeed, previous studies have reported specificity ranging from 50 to 67.6% and sensitivity of 86.5% (73,76,78).

Inoue and colleagues(79) , in their multicenter study of 105 eyes with type 1 CVN, found that the sensitivity of OCTA alone was 66.7%, identical to that of FA, and that this sensitivity increased to 85.7% when combined with structural OCT. In addition, they found good agreement between OCTA and conventional multimodal imaging, reaching 94.9% for active and 90.5% for quiescent NVC.

These results were confirmed by other studies which found a sensitivity of 81% and a specificity of 100% with good agreement between OCTA assessors in the detection of quiescent CVNs

(78,80).

4.3.2. The different types of neovessels in OCTA

4.3.2.1. Type 1 or occult, subepithelial neovessels:

They represent the most common phenotype of exudative AMD. They are characterized by the development of a neovascular membrane of choroidal origin between Bruch's membrane and the EP.

The FO may find a grayish appearance of the central region, a slightly accentuated DSR, sometimes hemorrhages, and exudates if the evolution is prolonged. FA shows minimal, initially irregular hyperfluorescence, with poorly defined late-stage diffusion, associated with small pinpoints of hyperfluorescence. Indocyanine green angiography (ICG) is more precise, rendering NVCs visible as well as their origin and ramifications. OCT B-scan usually shows a raised PE, associated with DSR and/or intraretinal edema(69).

On OCTA, NV type 1 appears as a pathological hyper-signal lesion beneath the EP at the level of the segmentation passing through the choriocapillaris. (Figure 37)

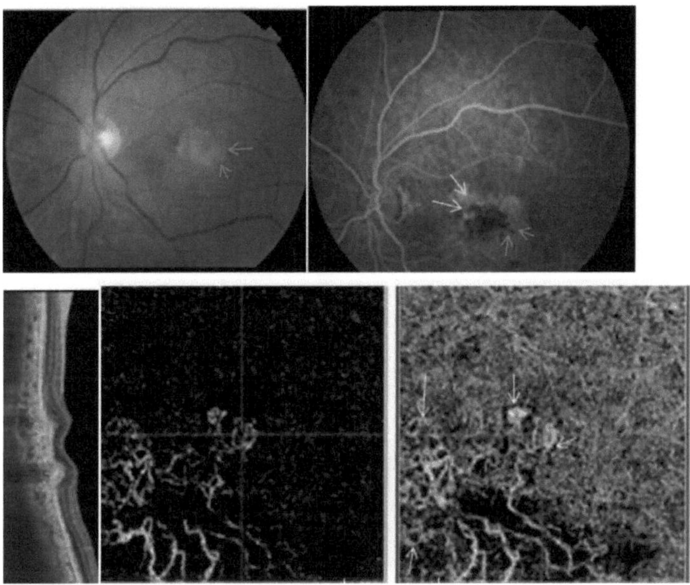

Figure 37: OCTA and NVC type 1 in OCTA.
Exudative AMD in a 65-year-old woman(A) FO: neovascular membrane with two punctiform hemorrhages (blue arrows). AF (B): peripheral heterogeneous macular hyper fluorescence (yellow arrows). OCT (C): hyperreflective fusiform thickening below the PE. OCTA of the choriocapillaris shows the presence of a neovascular network with branches emerging in all directions (jellyfish shape) with large-calibre vessels (red arrows) and peripheral capillary branches in the form of loops (white arrows).

Kuehlewein L et al (81) distinguished 3 patterns of high-flow lesions sharing common microvascular features:

- ***medusa*** pattern: vessels radiating in all directions from the radiating in all directions from the center of the lesion

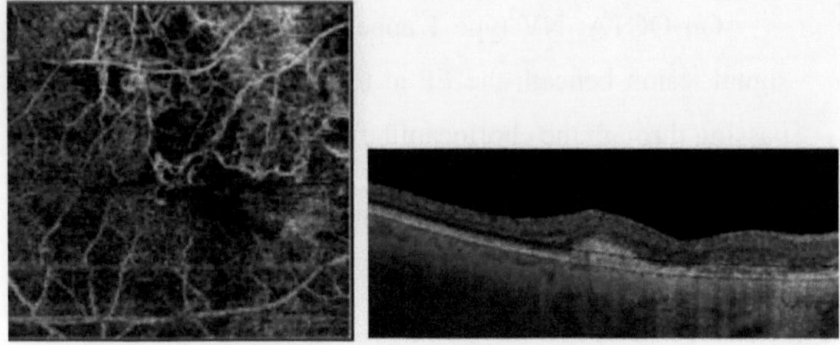

Figure 38: Medusa-shaped type 1 CVN

- ***The*** "seafan ***pattern" coral appearance***: where the main vascular trunks follow only one direction

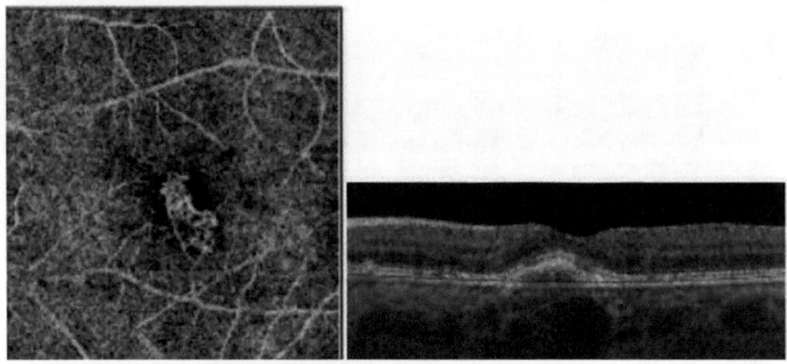

Figure 39: Coral-shaped CVN type 1

- **Undifferentiated appearance**<< indistinct pattern ": does not correspond to any of the preceding morphological patterns

A dark peri-lesional halo is often present, explained by alterations in choriocapillaris vascular flow, and identification of the feeder vessel is sometimes possible(82). The characteristics of type 1 CVN on OCTA are summarized in the table.

4.3.2.2. Type 2 or visible, pre-epithelial neovessels:

They are less frequently observed, but functionally more significant. These are NVCs that cross Bruch's membrane, then pass through the EP into the pre-epithelial retinal space.

The FO may show a grayish subretinal elevation associated with DSR, OMC and sometimes subretinal hemorrhages.

FA shows localized, well-delineated hyper-fluorescence with an early onset, increasing in intensity and then extending beyond the initial limits during the sequence. This neovascular lacis has a bicycle-wheel or fan-shaped appearance(70).

Structural OCT objectifies the CVN as a hyper-reflective, pre-epithelial, fusiform thickening with more or less well individualized margins, posterior shading and associated with indirect signs of sub- and intra-retinal exudation(69,70,76,83).

On OCTA, NVC type 2 appears as a hyper-signal lesion in front of the EP, with fine, interconnected branches linked peripherally by a thin anastomotic arcade, and highlighted on segmentation in front of the EP, passing through the avascular areas of the outer retina and into the choriocapillary layer. A dark, perilesional halo is often found in the choriocapillaris(70,83,84)(Table 2).

For morphology, El Ameen A et al(84) proposed a description similar to that of type 1 CVNs by Kuehlewein L et al. The "seafan pattern" was then named "glomerulus-shapedlesion" and type 2 CVNs were thus described as "glomerules" or "medusas".

OCT-A also makes it possible to see all the branches from the feeder pedicles to their fine branches and the peripheral arcade without the masking associated with diffusions. The sensitivity of OCTA for type 2 CVN appears to be excellent, reaching 100% in some studies (70).

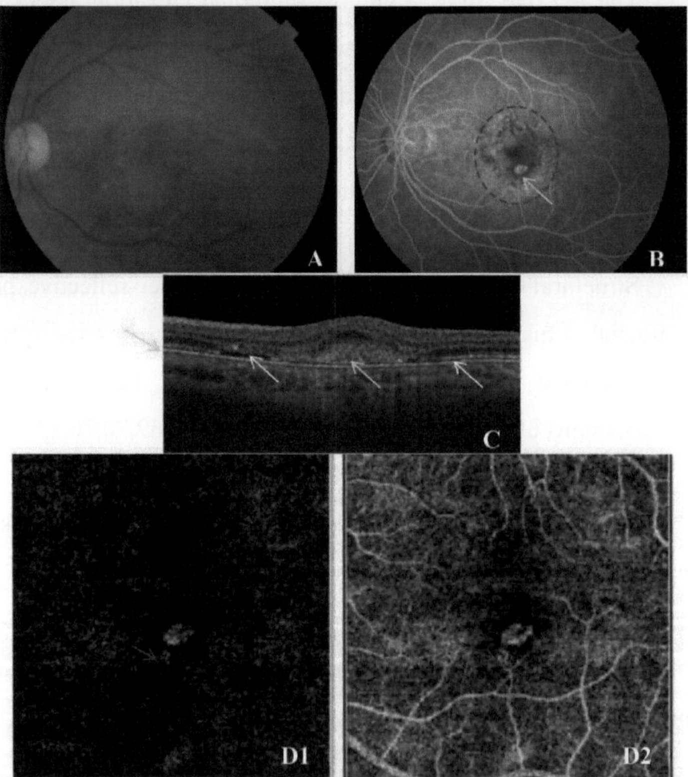

Figure 40: NVC type 2: OCTA appearance :
72 treated for AMD, consultant for abrupt OG AVB. Biomicroscopic examination showed the presence of macular serous drusen with yellowish inferior macular thickening(A)(red circles).FA (B) showed the presence of non-homogeneous macular hyperfluorescence, accentuated at the level of a rounded inferior lesion, reflecting the presence of a neovascular membrane(yellow arrow).OCT b scan (C) shows NVC as a fusiform thickening above the EP(yellow arrow)with interruption of the ellipsoid line (white

arrowheads).OCTA of the outer retina and choriocapillaris (D1/D2) shows the presence of a hyper-signal vascular lesion with the presence of a feeder vessel (red arrows) surrounded by a hypo-signal halo.

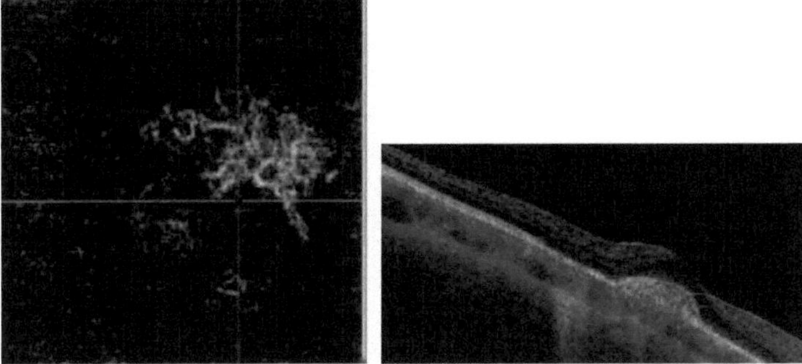

Figure 41: CVN type 2: jellyfish appearance on OCTA

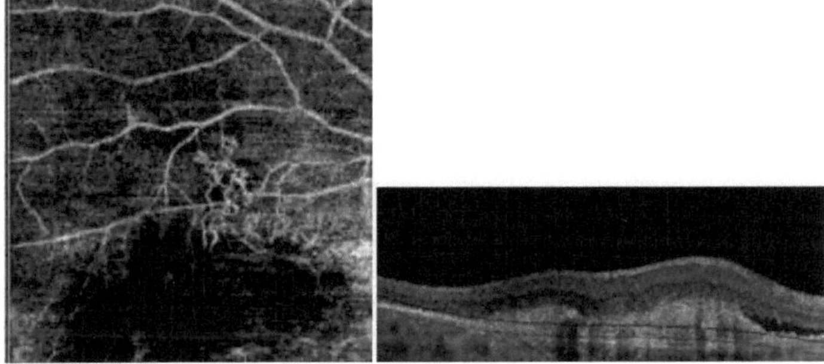

Figure 42: NVC type 2: glomerular appearance.
Note the presence of a feeder vessel (red arrow), with the various vascular branches pointing in the same direction.

4.3.2.3. Type 3 neovessels, or chorioanastomoses, are the most common type of neovessel.

retinal :

Often described as *retinal angiomatous proliferation.* This is a particular form of neovascular AMD, evoked by a macular functional syndrome with a rapid, acute drop in VA, associated with metamorphopsia.

The initial origin of the lesion is still debated, but most authors currently agree that the initial localization is retinal, with progressive extension under the PE(85).

The FO often finds small intra- or preretinal hemorrhages associated with the presence of a small, right-angled venule in the vicinity. This type of CVN frequently occurs in the context of reticulated pseudodrusen.

FA shows a juxta-foveal *hot spot* with localized and intense early hyper-fluorescence with rapid diffusion due to intra-retinal edema. Cystoid logettes and DSR are associated.

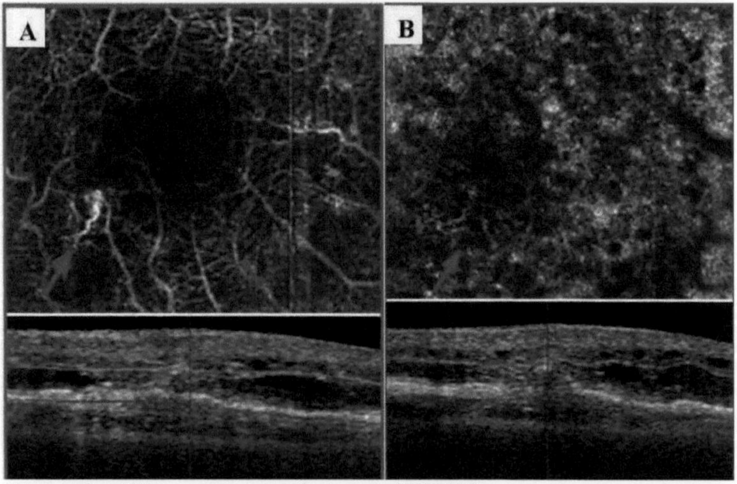

Figure 43: OCTA appearance of a type 3 CVN (54).

A: segmentation passing through the outer retina. At the level of the outer retinal segmentation, there is a small tuft-shaped high-flow lesion (red arrow). B: segmentation passing through the choriocapillaris. A greyish lesion in the form of a glomerular lesion is visible (red arrow).

ICG is the gold standard. Within a hypocyanescent EPD (dark background), it highlights the anastomosis comprising a retinal arteriole, a venule and a small cluster of deep NVCs with progressive diffusion(56). Structural OCT shows EP effraction, intra-retinal hyper-reflectivity and thinned choroid. Edema is often prominent in the vicinity of the anastomosis zone (56,85).

In OCTA, type 3 CVNs seem to have their own characteristics, unlike type 1 and 2 CVNs where the various aspects do not seem to be type-specific (table 2).

Firstly, recent OCTA studies reinforce the hypothesis of the initial retinal location of the lesion (86,87). NVC type 3 thus corresponds to an intra-retinal anastomosis originating in the deep plexus to form a tuft-like neovascular network in the normally avascular outer retina, which may extend to the EP. Consequently, the morphology of the neovascular complex differs according to the level of segmentation. A detailed examination of the segmentations at the level of the retinal plexuses and the choriocapillaris shows areas of hyper-signal (86).

- in the retinal plexi: angulation of the retinal capillary ;
- in the outer retina: *tuft-shape* appearance; detection at a very early stage, showing a hyperintense intra-retinal lesion with vascular flow.
- in the choriocapillaris: very dense and localized intense hyper-signal: *clew-likelesion(peloton)* .

Table II: OCTA signs of NVC types 1, 2 and 3

	NVC Type 1	**NVC Type 2**	**NVC Type 3**
Network ± detected	- Interconnected branches - Loops - Peripheral arch ± - Dark Halo peripheral±	- Interconnected offshoots + + + + +. - + loops - Peripheral dark halo + - Peripheral arch	Wick or tuft
Feeder trunk	± visible	Little detected +	Absent
Localization by flow superposition in cross-sectional OCT	High flow between Bruch and post-EP wall	Flux anterior to PE (PE effraction) in the outer retina	Intra-retinal and sub-PE flow
OCTA size *vs.* AF and ICG	Smaller	Similar	Stackable
Structural OCT	Exudative reaction	Exudative reaction	Major intra- and subretinal exudative reaction → under PE

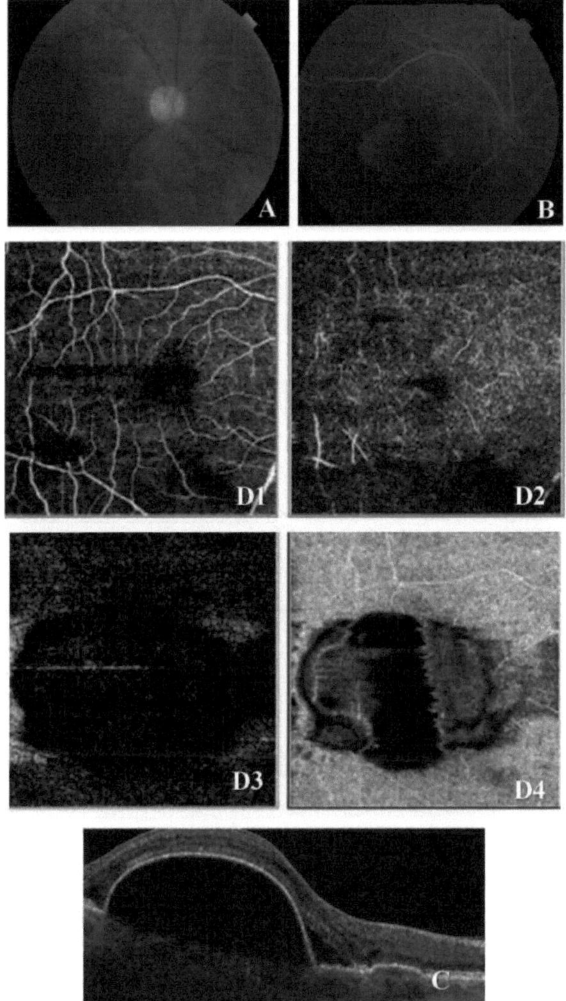

Figure 44: OCTA and exudative PED.
A 63-year-old woman with AMD consulted for OD BAV. Ophthalmological examination revealed a prominent centromacular lesion of yellowish appearance on the OF(A). The FA showed impregnation of the lesion by the dye, with no other visible abnormalities(B).The OCT B scan revealed a prominent EPD associated with a DSR with hyper-reflectivities of the EP in favour of the drusen. The ellipsoid line was also interrupted (C).
OCTA (automatic segmentation): shows the presence of projection artefacts due

to duplication of superficial vessels at the PVP level. PED translates into signal attenuation at the choriocapillaris without any obvious neovascular lesion.

4.3.3. Post-therapy follow-up

OCTA plays a key role in the initial assessment of exudative AMD. However, it can also be integrated into follow-up, if the hyper-signal is detectable and interpretable(88). After anti-VEGF IVT, quantitative and morphological changes in the neovascular lesion are observed on OCTA.

Quantitatively, a regression in neovessel size has been demonstrated. Muakkassa et al (89) reported a mean reduction of 23.6% in the area and 29.8% in the largest diameter of the neovascular lesion after treatment of naive NVCs.

Morphologically, a regression of flow within the vascular lesion has been demonstrated, with a rarefaction of the peripheral anastomotic arch and a less florid appearance, a progressive appearance of linear, voluminous, centrifugally arranged NVCs with a feeder trunk, and sometimes a decrease and/or disappearance of the peripheral dark halo (89,90).Some authors have also noted the presence of arterialization with extension of the feeder trunk, which could explain the chronicity of the pathology (91).

The kinetics of anti-VEGF action were also the focus of a number of studies, in order to pinpoint peak therapeutic efficacy and neovascular reproliferation phenomena. Taiichi Hikichi and colleagues (92) have shown that in exudative AMD treated with anti-VEGF, vascular density in the deep plexus and choriocapillaris decreases during treatment. Marques et al. found peripheral capillary loss from the lesion, vascular fragmentation and decreased vascular density at 7 days after IVT, followed by peripheral capillary reproliferation at one month. Huang et al.

(90) revealed a decrease in flow and lesion area at 2 weeks post-IVT with aflibercept, followed by reperfusion of some branches of the NVC at 4 weeks, 2 weeks before the appearance of exudative signs on multimodal imaging, suggesting earlier detection of rebound activity on OCTA than on structural OCT. Lumbroso et al (74) in their prospective study of type 2 NVC treated with anti-VEGF, found increasing vascular reduction of the lesion from the first day post IVT, reaching a maximum between 12 and 18 days. They also noted that the phenomena of vascular reproliferation and recanalization were observed between 28 and 35 days post-therapy, and that this evolution was repeated with each injection cycle. More recently, Miere et al (93) have suggested that NVCs never disappear, even with anti-VEGF treatment and the absence of SD-OCT activity.

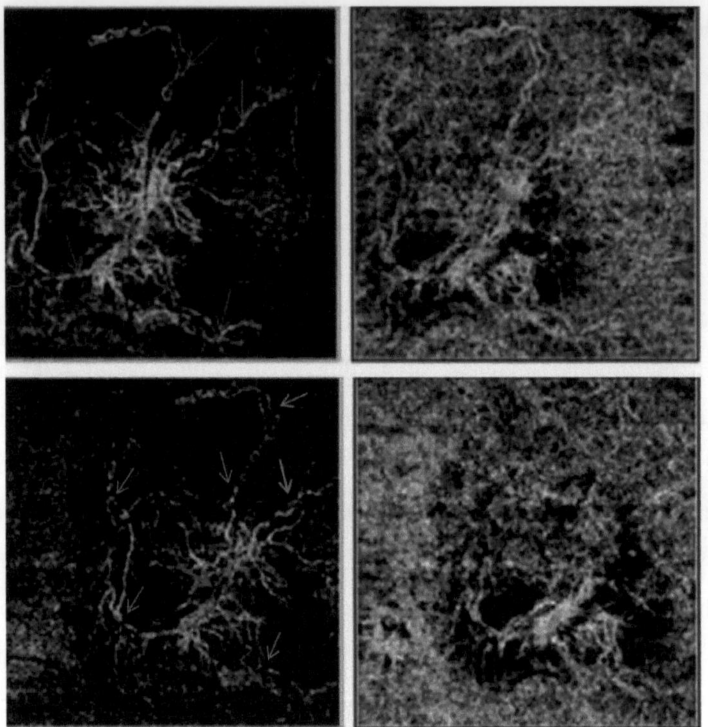

Figure 45: Exudative AMD and NVC type 2: post-therapeutic aspect. OCTA sections through the outer retina:
A1/A2initial appearance of NVC type2.B1/B2 aspect at D 7 post-treatment with IVT bevacizumab. Persistence of the central feeder trunk (red arrows) with regression of the caliber of peripheral branches and regression of peripheral loops and tortuosities.

In the late, scarring stage, subretinal fibrosis takes on a dead-tree appearance of hyper-signaling without interconnection between linear vascular pathways(94). Thus, recurrences and extensions of neovascularization following vascular remodeling may occur throughout follow-up, with the appearance of capillary buds at the periphery(93). OCTA appears to be an additional tool for determining the efficacy of treatment and for detecting possible recurrences. However, to date, there is no consensus on the follow-up of CVNs with OCTA, and the signs of activity detected by OCTA must be correlated with the usual signs of activity (DSR, haemorrhages, logettes)(88).

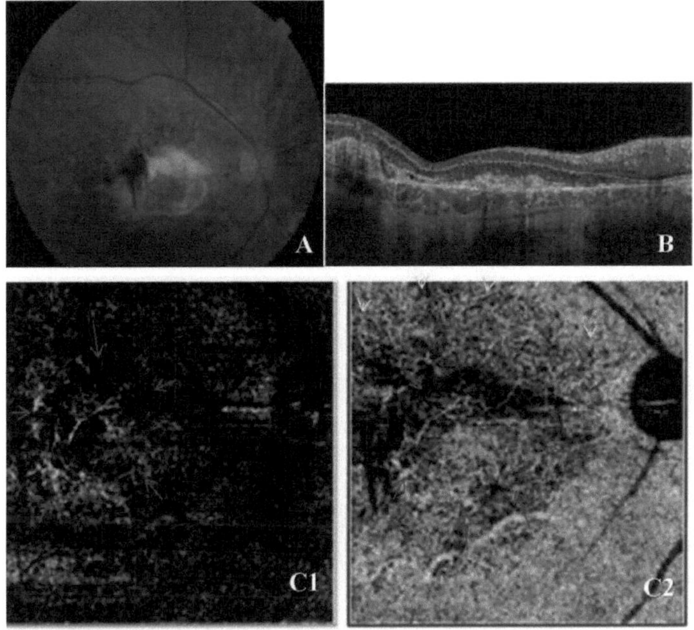

Figure 46: OCTA and fibro-glial scarring in neovascular AMD.
Neovascular AMD in an 82-year-old subject treated with anti VEGF IVT: Post-therapeutic appearance of a retinal fibrous lesion(A).OCT B scan shows scar hyper-reflectivity below the EP with no sign of activity and dedifferentiation of the various retinal layers, which become atrophic(B). On OCTA, we note the presence of a hyper-signal scar network with a dead-tree appearance (red arrows) (C1/C2) and no peri-lesional peripheral halo against a background of vascular rarefaction of the choriocapillaris (yellow arrowheads)(C2).

4.4. Limits :

Despite its many advantages, OCTA has certain limitations. First of all, the technique is patient-dependent, and the presence of low fixation and ocular saccades alters image acquisition quality.

Also, the threshold of detectable flow depends on the device used. As a result, some lesions may not be visualized because their blood flow does not reach the device's detection level(64). In addition, the best image resolution is obtained with the smallest windows (3x3), which limits the field of acquisition. Furthermore, OCTA does not reveal the rupture of the blood-retinal barrier, which is an important sign of neovascular activity(70,71,95).Finally, numerous artefacts and anatomical anomalies can alter interpretation (14,96,97):

- mirror artifacts, in which the retinal vessels are projected onto the EP ;
- signal blocking or attenuation artifacts, where the presence of very dense material or exudates can block the signal, causing retinal vessels to project at their level and mimicking the appearance of a CVN
- artefact due to the loss of the screen effect caused by the presence of the PE, where the choroidal vessels become visible, resulting in a hyperintense signal mimicking that of an NVC.

5. ANEURYSMAL NEOVASCULARIZATION TYPE 1 (POLYPOIDAL VASCULOPATHY)

Aneurysmal neovascularization type 1, formerly known as choroidal polypoidal vasculopathy (CPV), was first described in 1982 by Yannuzzi et al (98). It involves abnormal, branched vascularization of the inner choroid, associated with aneurysmal vascular dilatations that may be responsible for serous PED, and sometimes a true hemorrhagic picture.

It's a rare condition that mainly affects middle-aged black or Asian subjects. It is most often idiopathic, but may be secondary to various pathologies such as AMD, myopia, nevus... (99)

More recently, PCV has been integrated into the pachychoroid spectrum and renamed "neovessel type 1 with aneurysms"(100). It is a neovascular entity linked to a choroidal primum movens. It is characterized by frequent dilatation of the choroidal layers (Sattler and Haller) called "pachyvessels", associated with terminal aneurysmal dilatations called polyps. Ruptures of Bruch's membrane are sometimes found, as well as a type 1 neovascular network called branching vascular network (BVN) that develops between Bruch's membrane and the EP (figure 46)(99-102).

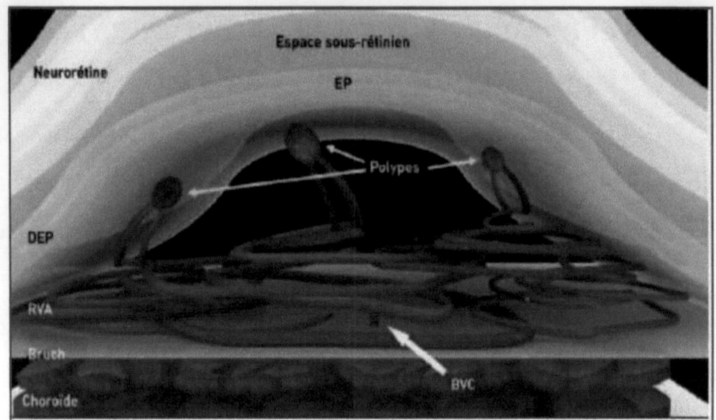

Figure 47: Pathophysiology of polypoidal vasculopathy.

Schematic representation of the relationship between polyps, the afferent vascular network (AVN), and choroidal vascular buds (CVB).

The etiology of PCV is unknown, but its predominance in black and Asian subjects suggests genetic factors. Mutations in the ATM gene may be involved in the development of PCV and macular telangiectasia. The majority of patients also had arterial hypertension.

Complementary examinations show characteristic images. Positive diagnosis is based essentially on ICG angiography.

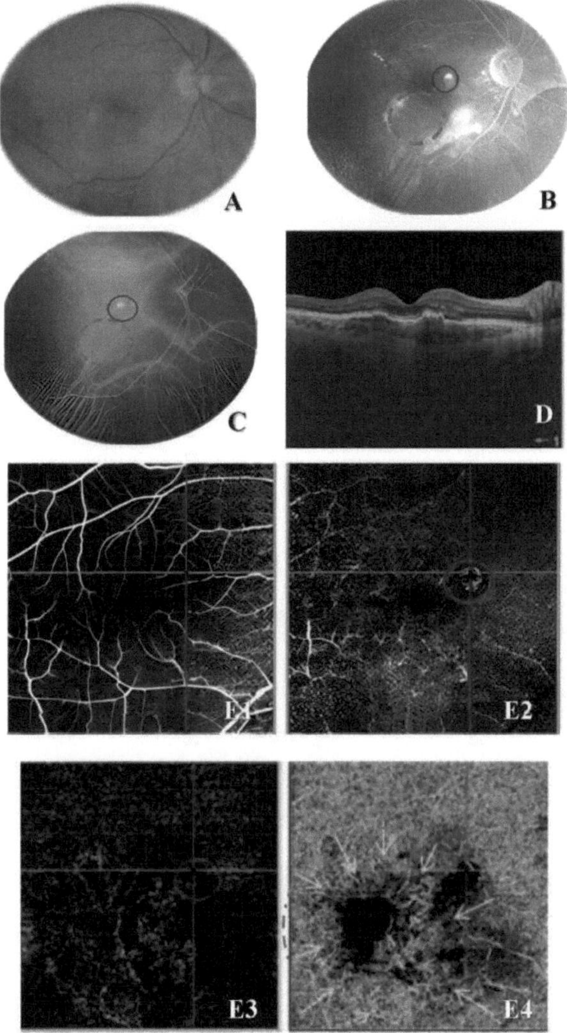

Figure 48: PCV without bleeding complications and multimodal imaging. 50-year-old woman: contralateral eye with subretinal hemorrhage(A).
The polyp: red circle: AF: non-homogeneous rounded hyperfluorescence, ICGA: hyper cyanescence with a hypo cyanescent peripheral halo; OCTA by sections passing through the top of the DEP: rounded hyper signal lesion with a hypo signal center and a hypo signal peri lesional halo.
BVN: green circle: hyper-fluorescent lesion on AF, hyper-cyanescent lesion on

ICGA and hyper-signal vascular network in the choriocapillaris with peripheral vascular branches (yellow arrows) and feeding choroidal vessels (red arrows).

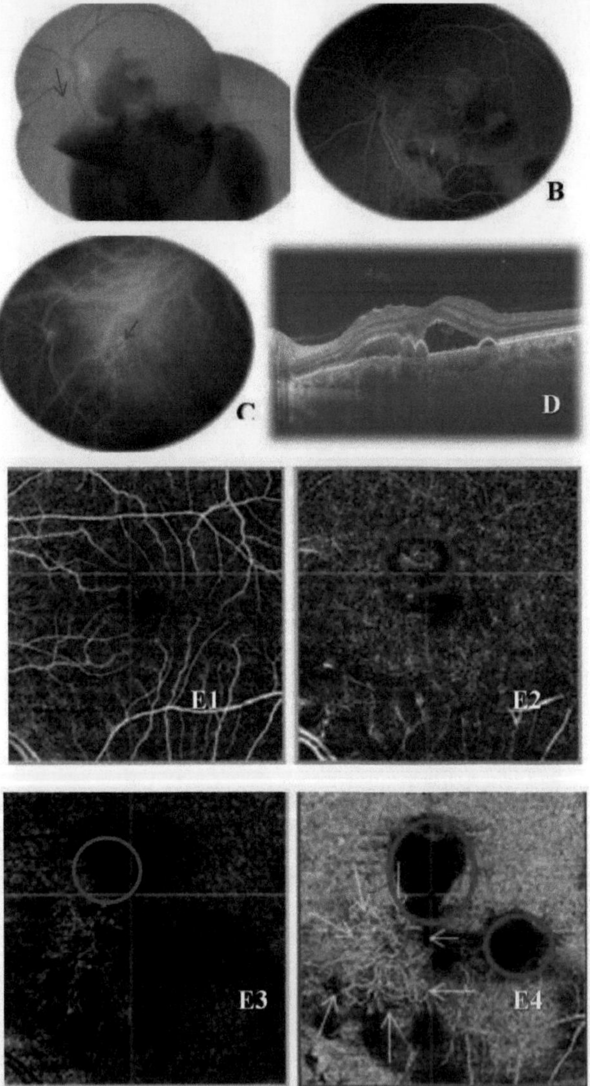

Figure 49: Subretinal hemorrhage secondary to CPV.
A 50-year-old woman with a history of retinal haematoma, the FO(A) showed a

deep sub-retinal haemorrhage of different ages occupying the posterior pole and inferior retina, with a deep orange-red lesion in favour of polypoidal lesion (red arrow), manifested on FA as a hyperfluorescent lesion smaller in size than that seen clinically, surrounded by a hypofluorescent halo(B).On ICGA(C), the polyp manifests as a peripheral non-homogeneous hyper cyanescence with a central hypo cyanescence of greater size than on AF.

OCT SD shows the presence of wavy, irregular EPDs (white arrows). Sub-retinal hemorrhage manifests as hyperreflectivity within hyporeflectivity secondary to a DSR.

OCTA revealed a normal appearance of the PVS(E1). The PVP showed a hyper-signal lesion with a hypo-signal halo in favour of the polypoidal lesion, which was individualized by a slice through the top of the EPD(E2). The BVN showed an irregular hyper-signal medusa head network (yellow arrows).The EPDs showed a-signal lesions in the CC due to the masking effect(E4).

Clinically, PCV is responsible for red-orange peri-papillary and inter maculo-papillary nodules associated with PED, intraretinal haemorrhage or haematoma and numerous exudates (Figure 47.48) (100). To date, there is no universally accepted definition of this condition, and multimodal imaging remains of great interest.

5.1. AF aspect of mail order :

The a VPC is characterized during the angiographic sequence by the appearance of aneurysmal-looking dilatations, progressively staining with retention, with little or no diffusion at the late stage. Occasionally, the dye disappears or is diluted at the end of the sequence. These polypoidal lesions are often associated in AF with a picture similar to that of occult neovessels, with heterogeneous, ill-defined hyper fluorescence, explained by the existence of an abnormal choroidal network or by occult neovessels complicating or associating with polypoidal dilatations. These lesions may be masked by haemorrhages collected on the neurosensory retina or under the pigment epithelium.

5.2. ICG angiographic appearance of VPC :

ICGA is traditionally considered the gold standard for diagnosing PCV, visualizing polypoidal dilatations in the form of hyperfluorescent lesions that are rounded in the early stages, giving a "grape cluster" appearance, and may persist in the late stages. Attenuation of the fluorescence of these lesions may be observed, leading to a wash-out phenomenon. BVN is visualized as a hyper-fluorescent plaque, observed from early on, and sometimes at late stages (figure 47.48). In contrast to AMD, the main differential diagnosis, ICGA also reveals choroidal hyperpermeability in PCVs(103,104).

5.3. Mail order in OCT :

B-scan OCT is an essential tool for diagnosing and monitoring PCV. Polyps are seen as moderately hyper-reflective, rounded lesions within a PED. The latter is marked, dome-shaped and often has steep edges. The B-scan OCT also shows a "double layer sign", characterized by irregular but flat uplift of the hyper-reflective EP, corresponding to the BVN. It also shows thickening of the choroid with remodelling that may be masked depending on the extent of the EP and/or intraretinal haemorrhages (Figure 47 D/48D)(100,105,106).Pachychoroidopathies are defined by dilatation of the "pachyvessel" choroidal vessels, structural remodeling with loss of the "**mosaic**" appearance, associated with a pathological increase in choroidal thickness compressing the choriocapillaris. All these lesions are well individualized in PCV, classifying it within the spectrum of pachychoroidopathies (100,102,105,107,108).

5.4. OCTA mail order :

For OCTA, its major advantage for PCV lies in the detection of the abnormal choroidal network and its location in relation to the EP, unlike polyps which are rarely visible due to the irregularity of their blood flow (99,109,109,110). Indeed, various studies have noted that with OCTA, the BVN detection rate is excellent (77.8 - 100%) and may be higher than with ICGA, whereas for polyps, the detection rate is heterogeneous (17 - 92%) and lower than with ICGA (103,104,111,112).

5.4.1. Appearance of polyps on OCTA:

OCTA enables segmental analysis of the different layers, as the polypoidal lesion is not located in the same plane, thus visualizing, at the level of the choriocapillaris segmentation, the abnormal BVN choroidal network as a hyper-signal lesion. In most cases, polypoidal lesions appear as round hypo-signal structures without flow, or as round hyper-signal structures with flow surrounded by a hypo-signal halo.

San Seong and colleagues classified the appearance of polyps on OCTA sections into 3 types:

- **the halo type** with high flux density surrounding the dark inner circular cavity and periphery
- **vascular network type** similar to BVN
- **the rosette type** with high flux density surrounding the irregular internal dark cavity and periphery(112)

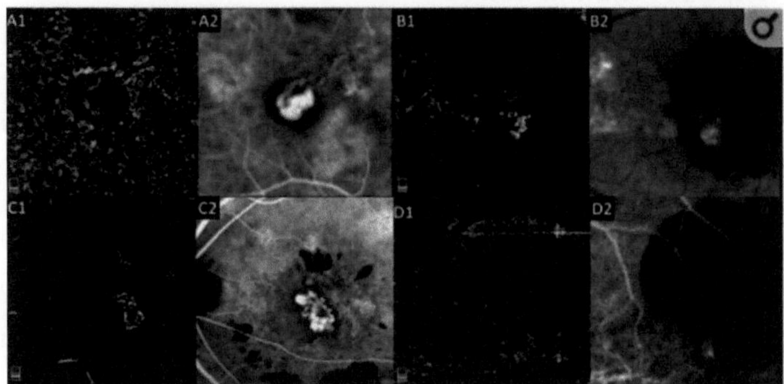

Figure 50: Comparison of polyps with different vascular patterns by OCTA and ICGA(111).
Case A/D: OCTA of the outer retina shows the polyp as a halo (A1/D1). Case B: OCTA of the outer retina shows the polyp signals as rosette B1. (B2) corresponds to its appearance in ICGA. Case C: OCTA of the outer retina shows the polyp as a hyper-signal similar to a vascular network (C1). C2 corresponds to its ICGA appearance.

The absence of a decorrelation signal within the polyp does not mean that there is no blood flow, but rather that the flow characteristics do not meet the OCTA detection criteria:

- Either the signal is attenuated by the PE
- Either the flow characteristics are undetectable: flow too low,

turbulent flow, flow circulating only at the periphery of the polyp, or there is hyalinization of the polyp with obstruction of the lumen after treatment (111-114). The detection of polypoidal lesions also depends on their size, and small polyps are difficult to detect by OCTA(101,115). Moreover, polyps are smaller on OCTA than on ICG. This could be explained either by impregnation and diffusion phenomena, which make it difficult to measure polyp boundaries on ICG, or by hyalinization of the vascular wall of polyps, with narrowing of its lumen.

5.4.2. Abnormal choroidal vascular network on OCTA:

the abnormal choroidal network, characterized by linear blood flow, is clearly detected by OCTA (detection rate between 55 and 100×)(116). These high-flow vessels are recognized at Bruch's membrane, as evidenced by histopathological studies. BVN complex flow is detected at an average of 28.6 µm below the PE reference plane, as proposed by a recent OCTA-guided study by Chi and colleagues(110). Various BVN patterns have been highlighted, such as the "Sea-Fan", tangled and jellyfish-head appearance(111)(117).

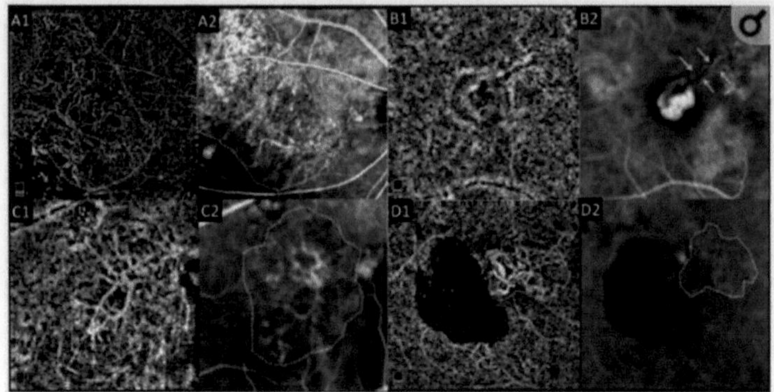

Figure 51: Comparison of BVN with different vascular models by OCTA and ICGA(111).
Case A: BVN in the form of a sea-fan (A1/OCTA aspect A2/ICGA aspect). Case B: BVN in the form of a feeder vessel and a draining vessel (yellow arrows) (B1/OCTA aspect/B2: ICGA aspect). Case C: BVN in the form of a medusa (C1 OCTA appearance/C2: ICGA appearance). Case D: BVN in tangled form (D1: OCTA appearance/D2: ICGA appearance).

Manual adjustment of the segmentation improves the chances of detecting polyps or the BVN. Indeed, OCT A-section images have shown that the BVN generally resides between the PE and Bruch's membrane, whereas polyps are located on a more anterior and variable plane. In addition, the low polyp flow and therefore low signal in OCTA may reduce polyp detection. Consequently, BVNs are a more essential feature than polyps for the diagnosis of PCV in OCTA(101,110,114,115,117).

Certain conditions limit the detection of BVN and polyps in OCTA: bulky PEDs especially as polyps reside at the top of PEDs, extra-macular polyps with haemorrhage or exudation, massive organized blood with exudation and finally polyps without significant branched vascular networks(108,110(99,109).

Consequently, OCTA is by no means a substitute for ICGA in the assessment and detection of PCV, and is incorporated into the multimodal workup (103,104,118).

6. CENTRAL SEROUS CHORORETINOPATHY AND OCTA

Central serous chorioretinopathy (CSRC) is a chorioretinal pathology characterized by a DSR of the posterior pole, linked to the passage of fluid from the choroid via a zone of low resistance, known as the leak point, which testifies to a microalteration of the PE. The choroid is the site of vasodilation and hyperpermeability, leading to thickening. Thus, CRSC falls within the recently defined group of pachychoroidopathies, comprising: isolated pachychoroid, pachychoroid-associated epitheliopathy, CRSC/diffuse retinal epitheliopathy (DRE), pachychoroid-associated type 1 neovascularization and PCV(108).CRSC is usually idiopathic. It is bilateral in 20 to 40% of cases and most often asymmetrical(119).This pathology encompasses several different clinical forms. The acute form is characterized by a DSR that often resolves spontaneously, in 3-4 months, with a good visual prognosis(120).The chronic form, also known as ERD, is defined by a duration of more than 4 to 6 months, during which the DSR persists or relapses, leading to retinal alterations, mainly of the photoreceptors and multifocal alterations of the EP, resulting in a progressive decrease in VA(121).Classically, the functional signs of acute CRSC include blurred vision, relative central or para-central scotoma, metamorphopsia, hyperopia, moderate dyschromatopsia, micropsia and reduced contrast sensitivity.

Type 1 choroidal neovascularization may complicate the disease. It occurs mainly during the course of chronic CRSC, with a frequency varying from 4% to 15% of cases according to studies(122-124).

6.1. CRSC: multimodal imaging :

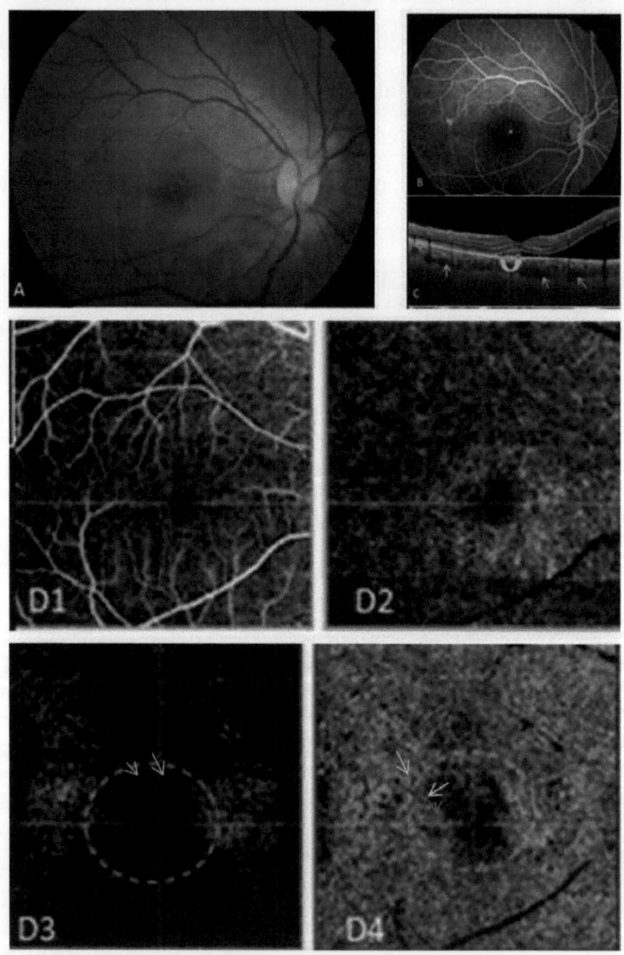

Figure 52: Acute CRSC and OCTA :

A 28-year-old woman. the FO(A): DSR involving the macula. the AF(B):diffuse alterations of the EP with a supra-macular vanishing point with duster-like diffusion of the dye (red arrow).OCT SD(C): a polylobed DSR with an irregular roof due to the presence of hyper-reflective material (blue arrow) with localized EP (yellow arrow), in addition to abnormal dilatation of the choroidal vessels (white arrows).OCTA sections show a normal-looking PVS (D1), hyper-signal perifoveal vessels in the PVP (D2), dark hypo-signal areas in the outer retina and choriocapillaris (green circles) (D3/D4) with dark spots in the choriocapillaris (green arrows).

At the FO, acute CRSC is characterized by the presence of one or more well-circumscribed DSRs, associated or not with mostly small PEFs and PE alterations (Figure 51/52). Chronic CRSC is associated with multifocal alterations of the PE, sometimes taking the form of "gravitational flows" (Figure 56)(125).in the case of acute CRSC, early FA shows focal or multifocal hyper-fluorescence with diffusion from one or more leakage points. Dye diffusion may then take on an "ink blot" or "feather duster" appearance. In the late stage, it shows inhomogeneous filling of the DSR(s) (figure 51B/52 B). In chronic CRSC, the hyper-fluorescence is more diffuse and inhomogeneous, reflecting the window effect associated with areas of retinal damage (figure57)(122). ICGA reveals anomalies that are highly characteristic of CRSC. In the early stages, it shows delayed filling of the choroidal arteries and choriocapillaris, abnormally dilated choroidal veins in the vanishing point zones, and areas of maximum multifocal hyper-fluorescence in the intermediate and late stages, it can show persistent hyper-fluorescence due to impregnation of the inner choroid, a wash-out of the large choroidal vessels, or a centrifugal evolution of the hyper-fluorescence in the intermediate phase, giving the appearance of a hyper-fluorescent late ring (figure

55 D)(125,127).ICGA may also show punctiform hyperfluorescence in the intermediate and late phases, reflecting choroidal hyperpermeability and choroidopathy(128).

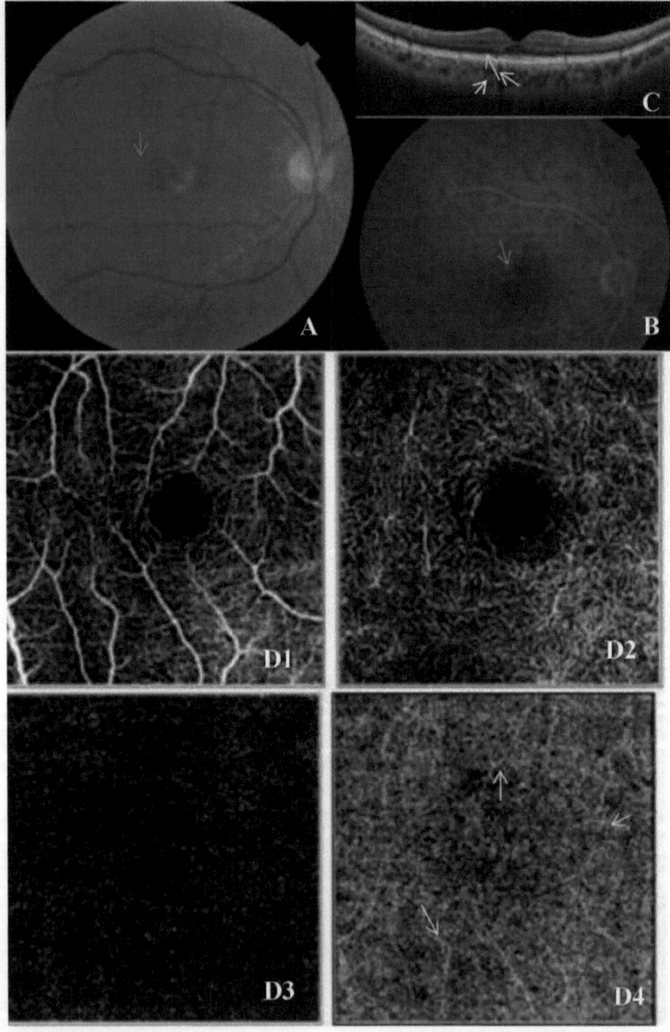

Figure 53: OCTA and adelphic eye anomalies in acute CRSC.

(A) :FO :supra-macular EP alterations.(B) :supra-macular hyper-fluorescence without window diffusion secondary to EP alterations.(C) : OCT SD choroidal vessel dilatation (white arrows) with EP irregularities (yellow arrows) and ellipsoid line interruption (red arrow).D1 :OCTA PVS :normal appearance. D2 :OCTA PVP/ widening of the ZAC with rupture of the perifoveal anastomotic circle (blue circle).D3 :normal appearance of the outer retina. D4:alterations in the capillary bed of the choriocapillaris with areas of hypo signal secondary to hypo-perfusion (red arrowheads) with peripheral capillary dilatation (yellow arrows).

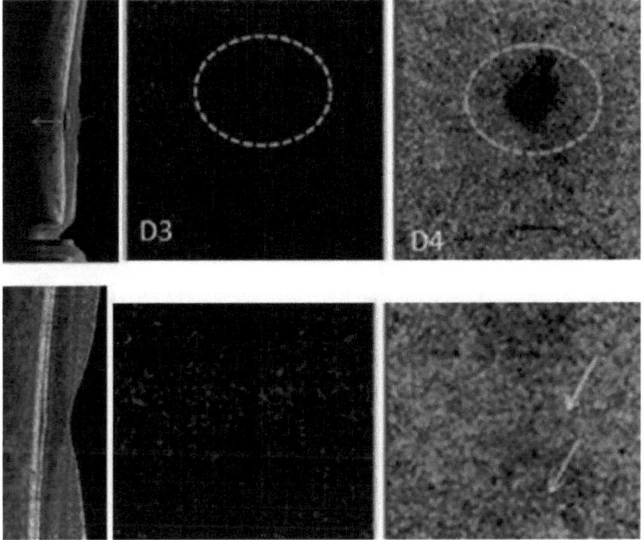

Figure 54: OCTA of the Choriocapillaris before and after resolution of the DSR during acute CRSC.
After resorption of the DSR, we note the persistence of hypo signal areas with the presence of hyper signal areas of hyper flow with vascular dilatations.

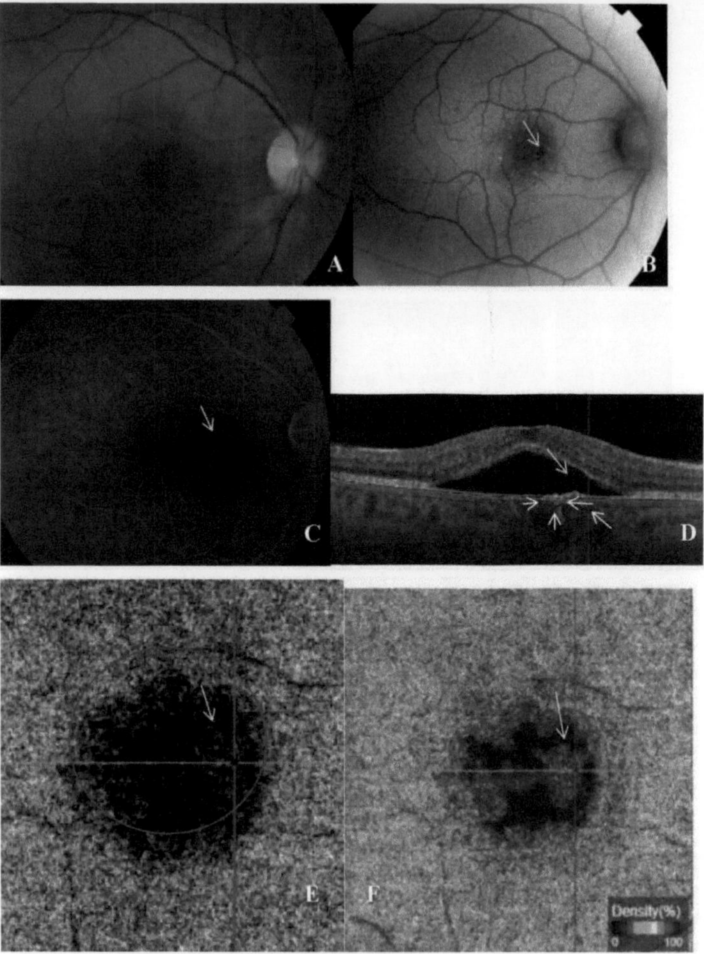

Figure 55: Choriocapillaris leak point in OCTA.

FO: Acute CRSC in a 40-year-old man(A). Auto fluorescence (B) shows the presence of hypo auto fluorescence corresponding to the leakage point objectified on FA(C) (yellow arrows).OCT B slice (D) scan passing through the leakage point revealed an irregular EPD (yellow arrow) above choroidal vascular dilatations(white arrows).The OCTA section of the choriocapillaris(E) shows the presence of the dark zone with vascular dilatations corresponding to the angiographic leak point.Vascular density mapping of the choriocapillaris(F) shows an intermediate density corresponding to dilated vessels within the low density associated with masking secondary to DSR.

For OCT B-scan, it classically shows in the CRSC:

- one or more DSRs, usually regular, in the form of hyporeflective uplift. This DSR may be associated with hyper-reflective subretinal deposits that may be complicated by subretinal fibrosis, and in around 70% of cases with photoreceptor elongation(125,129,130).
- A PEF, in more than 50% of cases, single or multiple, associated or not with a DSR and/or an angiographic leak point. It can be visualized as domes or irregular undulations of the PE, called "FIPED" (flat irregular pigment epitheliumdetachment), and most often located opposite areas of choroidal vascular anomalies observed on ICG(125,127,131).
- Thickening of the entire choroid (> 400µm) localized in areas of hyperpermeability visualized on ICGA. This thickening is associated with dilatation of the large choroidal vessels (Haller's layer) and thinning of the inner choroidal layers (Sattler's layer and choriocapillaris) (122,126,132,133). Dilated choroidal vessel walls may appear hyper-reflective in chronic CRSC, probably due to tissue remodelling(125).

The OCT B-scan can also show :

- PE abnormalities in the form of elevation at the leak point in the case of acute CRSC, or in the form of micro-tears, hypertrophy or atrophy in the case of chronic CRSC(134).
- Retinal abnormalities, generally found in chronic forms of

CRSC, such as hyper-reflective deposits in the outer layers, alteration of the outer segments of the photoreceptors, thinning or rupture of the outer layers; cystoid macular degeneration and sub-retinal fibrosis (125,127,135,136).

As far as OCTA is concerned, anomalies are mainly found in the choriocapillaris.

In the PVS, OCTA shows no abnormalities, whereas in the PVP, it can reveal vascular anomalies such as capillary dilatation and rupture of the perifoveal anastomotic ring.

In the outer retina, OCTA shows abnormal flow, better visualized by manual segmentation (137). It also enables assessment of superficial macular vascular flow, and studies have noted that this flow is more reduced in patients with CRSC than in normal subjects. This reduction is directly correlated, in addition to macular thickness, with visual decline during this condition and is considered an indicator of the progression of macular degeneration (138).The choriocapillaris is the main localization of abnormalities during CRSC. It allows visualization (136,137,139):

- Dark areas: correspond to areas of masking or hypo-perfusion, extensive or focal, hazy, poorly detectable. They are attributed to DSR, irregular plane DEP, hyper-reflective deposits or elongation of photoreceptor outer articles. These areas are present in 60% of CRSC(136).
- Dark spots: correspond to single or multiple, well-demarcated black spots where no flow is detectable. They are attributed to

domed, non-vascularized EPDs during acute SCRC and can be objectified alone or associated with dark areas(120,136). According to DEBAT et all ,in addition to PEDs, dark spots may correspond to sub-retinal deposits, choroidal cavitations, choroidal excavations and "lucencies", which on OCT B scan corresponded to a hypo-reflective sub-retinal cavity that matched the leakage point objectified on FA (138).

- Abnormal choroidal vessels: these correspond to areas of distinct, well-demarcated, high-flow, highly vascularized and entangled tangled patterns, i.e. abnormal dilatation of the choroidal vessels (136).these areas of hypo-perfusion in the choriocapillaris persist even after resolution of the DSR. This is explained by the fact that, during CRSC, the reduction in choroidal flow leads to congestion of the vessels in Haller's layer, resulting in compression of the choriocapillaris. Hypo-perfusion leads to reactive hydrostatic hyperpressure in a chronically hypoxic environment, resulting in impaired PE and the development of RSD (139,140).

Also, OCTA has shown a decrease in choroidal flow in acute CRSC. Various studies have looked for a correlation between the extent of areas of hypo-perfusion and progression to a chronic form or CVN. Indeed, according to MATET et all (141), areas of signal decrease increase with the duration of disease progression, with the extension of auto-fluorescence alterations and with the severity of chronic CRSC. On the other hand, GAWESKI et all found no correlation between the degree of choroidal damage and the patient's age, duration of symptom progression, initial retinal morphology and final visual acuity after remission of symptoms(142). Other studies have used OCTA to assess choroidal flow after treatment, which improves according to XU et all and FUJITA et all, with a gain in visual acuity(143).

6.2. CRSC complicated with NVC: multimodal imaging :

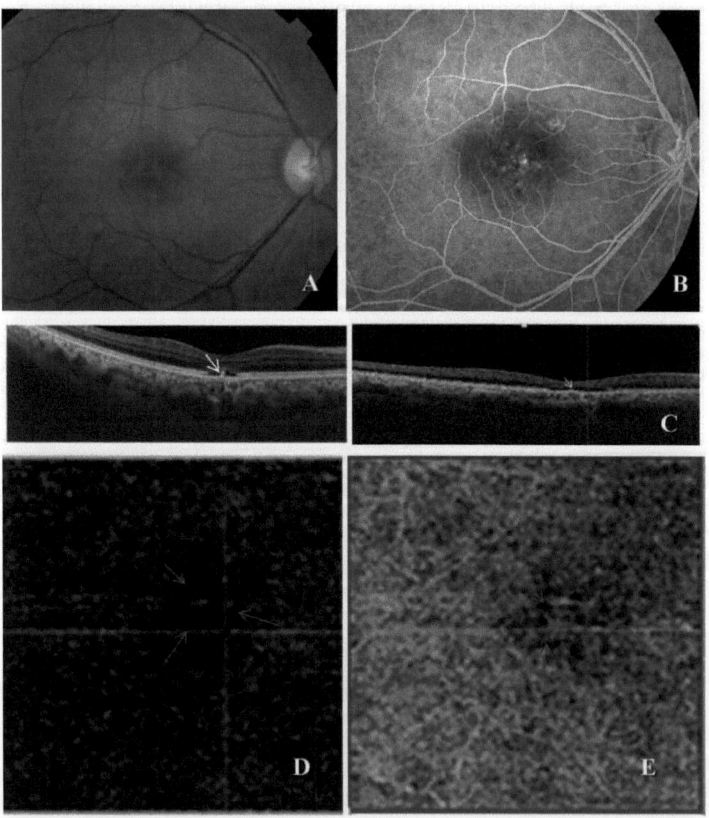

Figure 56: NVC figure complicating chronic CRSC.

55-year-old man followed for chronic CRSC on spironolactone:FO(A): diffuse alterations of macular EP. FA(B): diffuse inhomogeneous hyperfluorescence due to window effect. OCT B scan: presence of DSRs with hyperreflective content (C1/C2) (white arrows).OCTA: of the outer retina(D): presence of an abnormal hyper signal. OCTA of the Choriocapillaris (E) revealed the presence of an abnormal vascular laci with a tangled hyper-sigantic appearance and a peripheral hypo-signal halo (red arrows).

CVNs are a relatively rare complication of CRSC, with an incidence ranging from 2% to 9% (144).they occur mainly in chronic forms and FIPED-type PEDs(125,145)and are predominantly type1 CVNs(146).

However, the frequency of CVN in CRSC is probably underestimated, as its diagnosis is not always easy. In fact, the signs observed on multimodal imaging of chronic CRSC and type 1 CVN may be superimposable (144):

- At FA, PE alterations in chronic CRSC result in an inhomogeneous hyperfluorescence resembling the appearance of CVN type 1.
- On ICGA, the hyper-fluorescence of leaky spots at late time is sometimes difficult to differentiate from the late plaque characteristic of type 1 CVN. The presence of a neovascular laceration at early time is the most discriminating sign of CVN. However, this lacis is only observed in 50-60% of cases(145,147).
- On B-scan OCT, a DSR and/or intraretinal logettes can be seen in both chronic CRSC and type 1 CVN. In addition, FIPEDs have an appearance that may resemble a PED in type 1 CVN.

Nevertheless, a hyper-reflective EPD may be a sign of a neovascular complication, unlike a hypo-reflective EPD(105), and neovascularized FIPEDs appear thicker and wider than non-neovascularized FIPEDs(147).

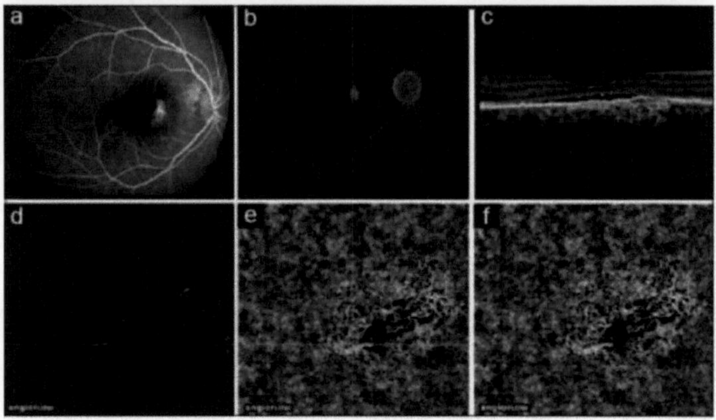

Figure 57: OCTA AND NVC complicating chronic CRSC (148).

A 48-year-old patient with chronic CSC with early (a) and late (b) phase FA showing dotted hyperfluorescence without progressive enhancement but who was diagnosed NVC by two experts according to BANSAL et all. SD-OCT slice (c) showed an irregular EPD with subretinal fluid accumulation. En face OCTA showed a neovascular complex, subtle in the outer retina (d) and prominent in the choroid (e). Automated segmentation visualized a larger, denser neovascular network (f).

OCTA, in chronic CRSC, can provide a useful element and be a high-performance examination for visualizing CVNs. Numerous studies have evaluated the prevalence of CVN on OCTA, with results ranging from 24.2% to 58% (136,144,144,147,149).

Some studies have demonstrated the superiority of OCTA over combined OCT/ AF/ICGA for the detection of CVNs in chronic CRSC, with better identification of their structures. Indeed, Bousquet et al(147) noted CVNs in 35% of irregular EPDs, whereas they were identified in only 19% of cases by multimodal imaging(150). OCTA has also been shown to visualize CVNs in FIPEDs in 24% to 42% of cases, and even in 90% of cases in some studies(136,144,147,151).

This NVC appears on OCTA, as in other pathologies, in the form of a hyper-signal vascular laceration, generally smaller in size than type 1 NVCs in AMD.

However, despite its greater sensitivity and specificity, OCTA can produce false positives, and irregular choroidal vascular laci could correspond to abnormally dilated choroidal vessels or NVC. For these reasons, some authors suggest comparing and contrasting OCTA findings with those of multimodal imaging before retaining the diagnosis of CVN complicating CRSC (120,136,147,148,152).

7. OCTA AND RETINAL VEIN OCCLUSIONS

Retinal vein occlusions (RVOs), which include central retinal vein occlusions (CRVOs) and retinal vein branch occlusions (RVOBs), are the 2ème leading cause of retinal vascular disease after DR, and their prevalence increases with age. They are due to the existence of an obstacle to venous outflow, leading to reduced perfusion and increased back pressure in the retinal circulation(153).their anatomo-functional prognosis is conditioned by the occurrence of 2 main complications: OM and/or retinal ischemia and its neovascular complications.

The diagnosis of RVOs is essentially clinical, with visualization of the classic tetrad: papilledema, venous dilatations, retinal hemorrhages and cottony nodules (Figure 60). Complementary examinations are used to classify RVOs as edematous, ischemic or mixed.

For many years, FA has been considered the reference examination for RVO. It confirms the diagnosis by showing the arteriovenous delay, specifies the clinical form and locates the contrast leak responsible for the RVO. However, this technique has several limitations linked to leakage or accumulation of contrast medium secondary to capillary hyper-permeability and perfusion defects, and ischemic signs are often obscured if edema or hemorrhage impede visualization of the capillary bed(154).

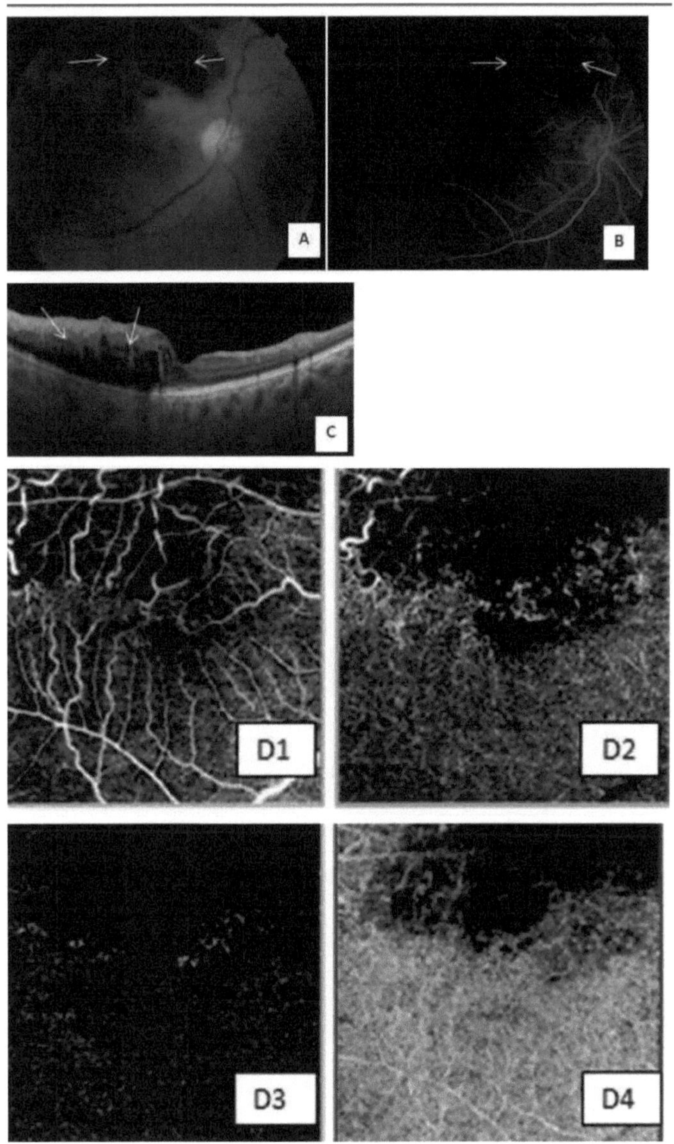

Figure 58: OBVR in multimodal imaging.
Superior temporal OBVR with Superficial(A)TAF retinal hemorrhages:

masking of large vascular vessels secondary to the presence of hemorrhages. SD OCT shows the location of the haemorrhages as hyper-reflectivity with posterior shading and localized macular thickening. OCTA shows the presence of large tortuous trunks in the PVS with capillary loss(D1).Signal loss secondary to the presence of haemorrhages is visible in the PVP(D2), outer retina(D3) and choriocapillaris(D4).

B-scan OCT has established itself as the reference examination for diagnosing and monitoring OM. It can confirm the diagnosis of RVO by showing haemorrhages in the oedema bullae, a characteristic sign of RVO (figure 60). It can also be used to suspect the vasogenic or ischemic nature of retinal thickening. In fact, in vasogenic OM due to rupture of the BHR, the damage is more likely to be in the outer retina, with the presence of numerous bullae, whereas in ischemic OM, retinal opacification is more extensive. However, the presence of edema or haemorrhages may prevent visualization of the ellipsoid zone(155).

Thus, the extent of ischemia and the assessment of its evolutionary risk remain a diagnostic and therapeutic challenge. In fact, in RVOs, non-perfusion generally progresses from the periphery to the center. Today, ultra-wide-field angiography, a new imaging technique, makes it possible to analyze the entire retinal periphery with a single image, to explore an area 3 times larger than with FA, and to facilitate assessment of the progression of peripheral non-perfusion (156).

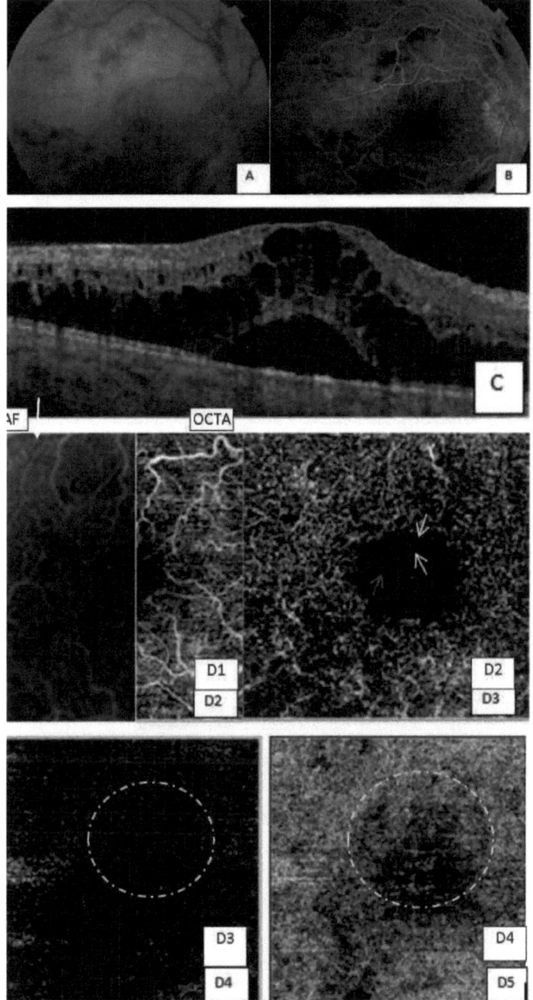

Figure 59: OCTA and edematous OVCR.

Fo: OVCR in a 38-year-old man (A).FA shows OVCR with peri-macular ischemia, with the presence of microaneurysms and peri-macular capillary tortuosity (B).OCT b scan of OCTA:cystoid OM with predominant logettes in the outer retina (white arrows) with DSR(C).Comparison between the appearance of the PVS in the AF and the OCTA shows greater enlargement of the ZAC in the AF, the limits of which are difficult to identify. The number of microaneurysms, a sign of ischemic maculopathy, is greater in the AF than in the OCTA(D1). In the PVP(D2), the cystoid spaces appear smaller on OCTA, depending on the level of the cut. Hypo-signal meshes (yellow arrows) separate a-signal spaces (red arrows) corresponding to cystoid logettes. In OCTA, the DSR is reflected by an attenuation of the signal visible in the outer retina (D3) and the choriocapillaris (yellow circles) (D4).

The recent advent of OCTA has opened up new diagnostic perspectives. It has been shown that in RVO, capillary occlusion more often affects the deep network than the superficial one(154). OCTA allows separate visualization of the two networks, which are superimposed and confused on FA. Thus, OCTA is currently considered a reliable, non-invasive examination for assessing the macular microcirculatory consequences secondary to RVO, with good correlation with FA, the reference examination, for assessing macular ischemic zones and microvascular remodeling(157-159).

In the macula, several abnormalities have been described(154,160,161). Compared with the adelphic eye, OCTA shows a widening of the ZAC, particularly in the PVP. It also shows an increase in para-foveal capillary non-perfusion and a decrease in para-foveal vascular density assessed by flow quantification software. In addition, it visualizes intra-retinal logettes better than structural OCT, and objectifies *shunting* between the superior and inferior vascular networks or at the papillary level (figure 61). All these anomalies may be present whatever the clinical form of the RVO and whatever its topography (OVCR, OBVR).

On the other hand, OCTA not only provides diagnostic elements for RVO, but also prognostic elements. Indeed, a quantitative correlation between macular capillary non-perfusion zones, parafoveal vascular density, ZAC widening and VA has been demonstrated, confirming that VA is dependent on several factors in addition to macular thickness(162-165).

It has also been demonstrated by OCTA that IVT of anti-VEGF and dexamethasone implants only stabilize macular perfusion and do not reperfuse the capillaries(166-168) (Figure 62).

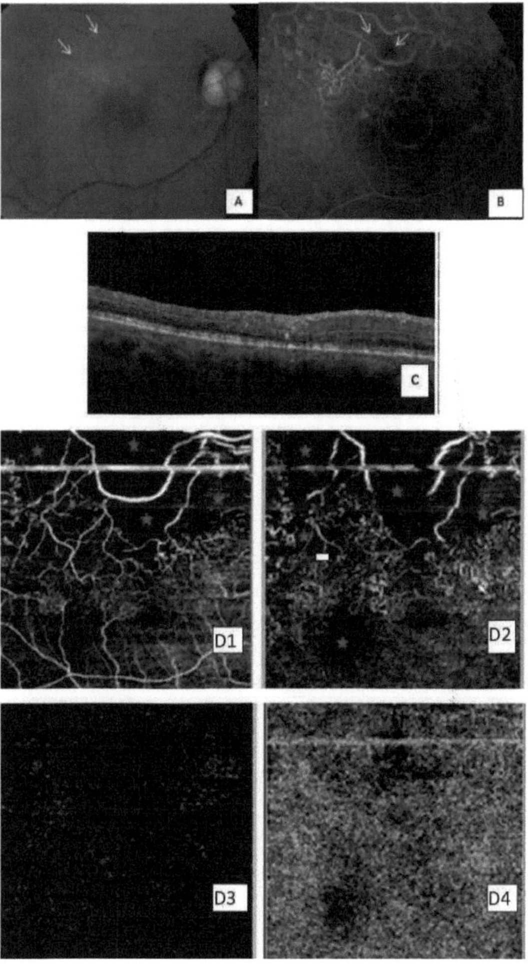

Figure 60: Venous-venous shunts in OCTA :
FO:superior temporal OBVR (presence of unhabited venous branch (white arrows))(A). FA: blockage of venous filling at the level of two venules (yellow arrows) with the presence of downstream venous collaterals (green arrowheads).Peripheral ischemia (red stars) with mixed maculopathy (red circle) (B). OCT B scan shows focal retinal thickening with dedifferentiation of the inner retinal layers, which appear hyper-reflective. OCTA(D1/D2/D3/D4) revealed areas of ischemia (red stars) that appeared more extensive in the PVP(D2) than in the PVS(D1) and compared with those seen in AF. The vascular tortuosities were more clearly visible than in AF (double blue arrow).OCTA made it possible to follow the path of the collaterality network in the PVS.The outer retina appeared normal(D4) and we also noted the presence of areas of choroidal ischemia(D5)with a decrease in capillary density in the PVP(D2).

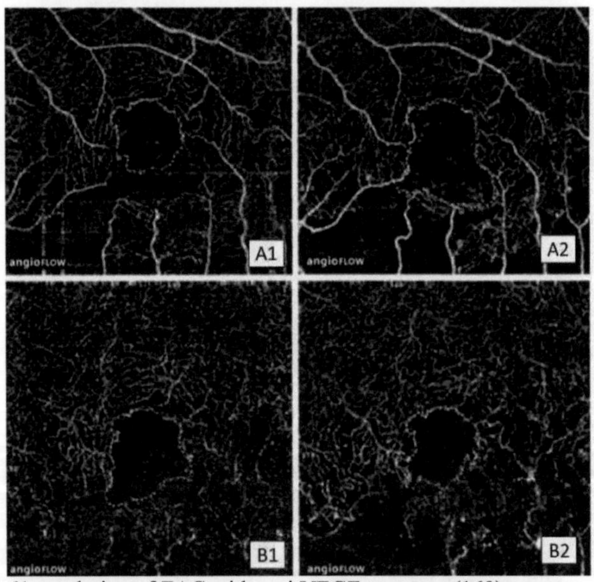

Figure 61: evolution of ZAC with anti VEGF treatment(169) :

The ZAC seen on OCTA in a patient with OBVR. (A1) Initial PVS (Bl)PVP 6 months after treatment. (A2) Initial PVP. (B2) PVP 6 months after treatment. The ZAC encircled by the yellow line was enlarged after treatment in the PVS.

As far as the retinal periphery is concerned, FA remains the reference examination for assessing the degree of secondary retinal ischemia. However, some OCTA devices, including our own, use automatic mosaic reconstructions to provide wide-field visualization and approach the surface explored by conventional angiography. A "wide field" of the retina is explored by mounting several 12 mm squares or 9 x 15 mm rectangles.

Several authors have studied the contribution of wide-field OCTA to the assessment of non-perfusion in RVO compared with ultra-wide-field AF, and have shown that OCTA enables "at-risk" non-perfusion territories to be detected with very good sensitivity and specificity (170,171). Visualization of non-perfusion territories of more than 3 papillary areas on wide-field OCTA is associated with the presence of retinal ischemia greater than one quadrant. This should lead to the performance of FA for a more formal diagnosis of non-perfusion(18,154,172).

In addition, a correlation between macular and peripheral vascular density has been demonstrated. Indeed, macular alterations observed on OCTA are statistically correlated with the presence of peripheral ischemia found on FA. When the vascular density of the deep capillary bed is less than 46%, there is a peripheral non-perfusion area of more than one quadrant in 66.6%, whereas it is only observed in 7.7% if density is greater than 46%(165,173).

Despite its great benefits, OCTA has certain limitations in RVO, especially for vascular density analysis, where artifacts can be numerous:

- in ischemic RVO, analysis of capillary rarefaction and calculation of macular vascular density may be masked by the presence of perivenular white (hyper-reflective on B-scan OCT), which will hamper visualization of the two retinal capillary plexuses
- in edematous OBV, analysis is also difficult in the presence of CMT or significant retinal hemorrhages
- In chronic OMs, most often associated with the secondary development of venous macroaneurysms, visualization of these vascular dilatations is not easy, probably due to the low flow inside the macroaneurysm(figure 63).
- In the case of wide-field OCTA, it can be a long and tedious process for some patients who have difficulty fixing the target.

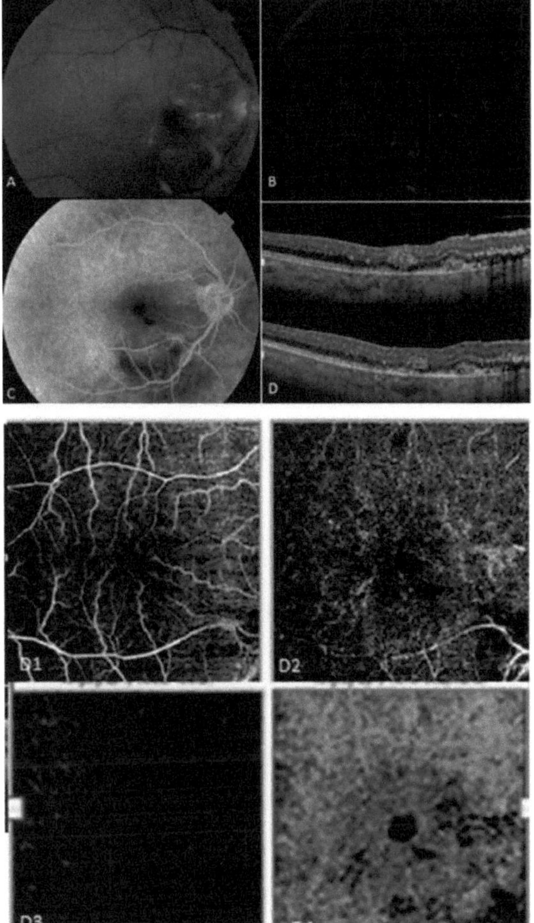

Figure 62: Venous macroaneurysm complicating retinal vein occlusion.

The patient was 53 years old. FO (A/B): a pigeon's nest macular hemorrhage with an exudative placard surrounding a whitish lesion opposite the inferior temporal arch, with amputation of the course of a vein opposite this lesion. AF(C) shows delayed venous filling opposite a macroaneurysm located at an arteriovenous crossing zone. OCT B scan (D): the macroaneurysm with thickening of the various retinal layers and hyper-reflective material corresponding to deep exudates. OCTA: hypo-signal lesions secondary to exudates, with rarefaction of peri-macular vascular density (D1/D2), which may be secondary to actual hypo-perfusion or masking due to hemorrhage.

Macroaneurysms appear in the outer retina and the choriocapillaris (D3/D4) in the form of an a-signal zone secondary to the absence of flow due to thrombosis or slowed or turbulent flow.

8. OCTA AND RETINAL ARTERIAL OCCLUSIONS

Retinal arterial occlusions (RAOs) are circulatory interruptions or slowdowns in all or part of the retinal arterial network. They are serious accidents, both visually, where they cause 60% of unilateral blindness with the risk of bi-lateralization, and in general, since they most often reflect suffering of the entire vascular system(174).

Depending on the site of obstruction, a distinction is made between occlusions of the central retinal artery (OACR) and occlusions of retinal arterial branches (OBAR). The evolution and functional prognosis are all the more serious when the occlusion involves a large trunk or a macular vessel. This pathology has two phases: acute and late.

In the acute phase, the diagnosis of OAR is usually straightforward. The FO finds ischemic whitish edema in the occluded territory, associated with a cherry-red macula appearance in the case of OACR, sometimes with visualization of the embolus responsible for the occlusion. FA confirms the diagnosis by showing delayed or absent arterial filling. However, AF can only explore and analyze the largest vessels, which may also be hampered by edema-induced light diffraction phenomena.

Structural OCT makes a major contribution to OAR. On the one hand, it confirms the diagnosis in total or subtotal forms, and on the other, it describes the anomalies of the different vascular plexi, consecutive to the different levels of retinal ischemia (174-176).Indeed, OCT shows retinal thickening and hyper-reflectivity of the inner layers secondary to PVS ischemia. It also reveals a hyper-reflective band in the inner nuclear layer known as acute para-central middle maculopathy (PAMM), a sign of ischemia of the PVI and PVP. In addition, it reveals a diffuse, hyper-reflective thickening of the inner and middle retinal layers, representing ischemia superficial and deep capillaries.

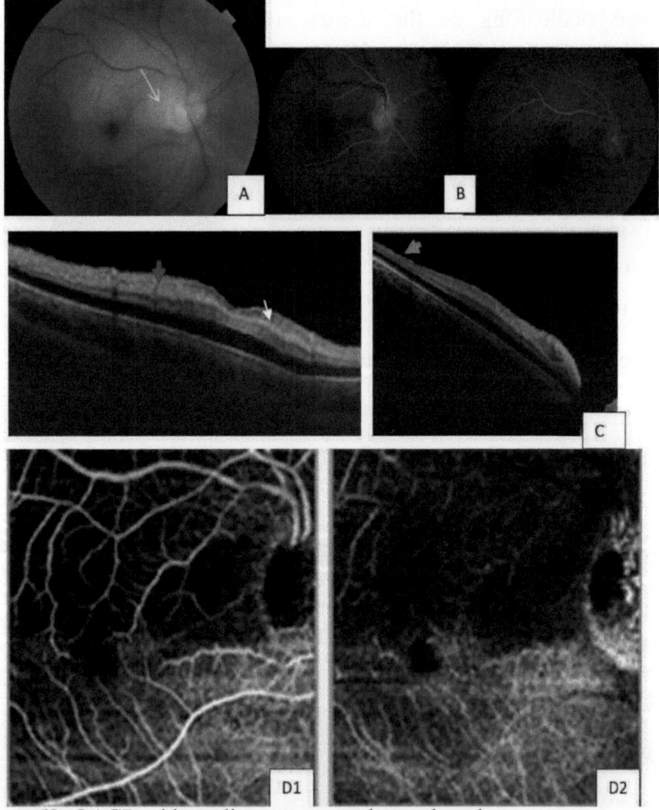

Figure 63: OACR with medium paracentral maculopathy.
FO (A) shows a cherry-red macular appearance with the presence of pale edema in the inter maculo-papillary area (yellow arrow) and ischemic appearance of

the temporal retina (red arrows).AF(B): delayed arterial filling with prolonged arteriovenous time and delayed filling of the superior temporal venous branch. OCT SD(C): thickening of the various retinal layers involving the inner layers of the retina (red arrows), predominantly inter maculo-papillary (yellow arrow), with a hyper-reflective bunghole (white arrow) indicating PAMM with peripheral retinal atrophy (green arrows). OCTA: disappearance of the supramacular retinal capillary bed at the level of the two vascular plexi (D1/D2) with persistence of large-calibre vessels at the level of the PVS (D1). conservation of the ZAC at the level of the two plexi.

OCTA enables us to better analyze the various plexi and pinpoint areas of ischemia without being hampered by diffraction phenomena caused by edema. Bonini et al found that whatever the form of occlusion, there is a decrease in perfusion of the PVS and PVP, corresponding to areas of inner retinal changes in OCT and areas of delayed perfusion in AF. This underscores the value of this technique in pinpointing and identifying the topography of the affected plexi and the limits of non-perfusion, a fact well demonstrated and confirmed by several other studies(177-182).

Indeed, Philippakis et al(181)suggested a greater susceptibility of the PVP in incomplete OARs. Baumal et al(177) have shown, in the case of OACR, a decrease in perfusion of the PVS and PVP, although the lesions are different where they noted a continuum between isolated lesions of the superficial plexus and combined and symmetrical lesions of the PVS and PVP. In OBAR, these authors noted that non-perfusion is more marked in the superficial plexus than in the deep plexus, and they found a well-defined decrease in flow and territory of ischemia downstream of the site of obstruction, with focal deficits in the territory of the occluded artery at the peripapillary level. On the other hand, compared with FA, OCTA has been shown to be more sensitive than FA in pinpointing the extent and magnitude of non-perfusion in OBAR(183).

In the late phase of OAR and after reperfusion, FA may show arterial narrowing with normalized fluorescein transit. B- scan OCT shows progressive atrophy of the inner retinal layers with less reflectivity than in the acute phase, associated with disappearance of ischemic edema(174). On OCTA, flow is again visualized in certain arterioles.

However, OCTA has certain limitations in SROs(183). In the case of complete occlusion, disorganization of the retinal layers may prevent proper segmentation and hence specific analysis. Also, in late phases, it is not easy to differentiate the different plexuses due to extreme retinal thinning. What's more, OACR is often associated with deep BAV and hence lack of fixation, leading to poor-quality imaging.

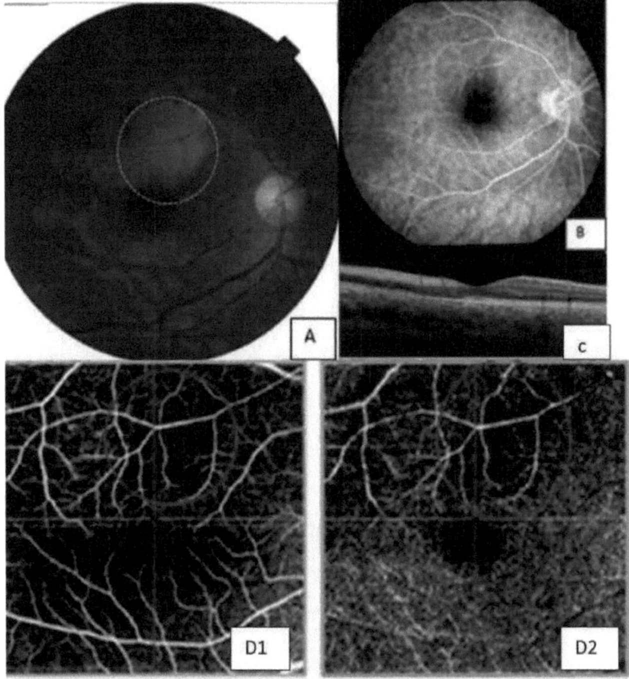

Figure 64: Retinal arterial branch occlusion.
12 YEARS: FO an area of supra-macular retinal ischemia (A: green circle). AF: delayed filling of a superior temporal retinal arterial branch showing caliber narrowing at its origin (yellow arrows) with downstream vascular dilatation(B). OCT SD(C): localized atrophy of the various retinal layers (white arrow), especially the inner layers, which appear hyper-reflective, with local interruption of the ellipsoid line(C)(red arrows).OCTA (performed after 48 hours of BAV): localized suprafoveal rarefaction of retinal vascularization in the PVS, with predominance of small-calibre vessels (D1); this hypoperfusion is more marked in the PVP, allowing visualization of the projection of superficial vessels against a background of ischemia (D2).

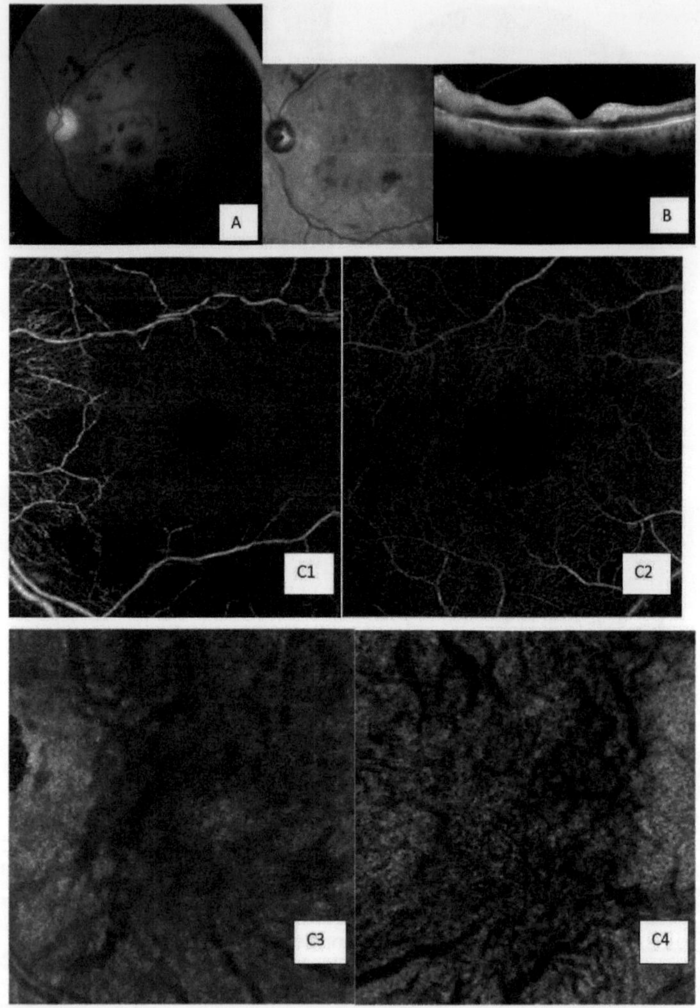

Figure 65: Combined occlusion of the central retinal artery and vein (184): A 69-year-old woman with abrupt OG AVB, FO shows papilledema with macular edema, venous tortuosity and patchy hemorrhages(A). OCT SD shows hyperreflectivity with retinal edema involving the inner layers of the retina(B). OCTA: capillary rarefaction with reduced flow in the PVS(C1) and PVP(C2) with no obvious involvement of the choriocapillaris(C3) and choroid(C4).

9. VARIOUS PATHOLOGIES

9.1. Angioid striae :

Angioid striae are folds in Bruch's membrane, first described by Doyne in 1889.these fissures occur on a fragile, thickened and calcified Bruch's membrane, with or without associated atrophy of the pigment epithelium and choriocapillaris.AS is a frequent cause of choroidal neovascularization. In 50% of cases, this pathology is associated with a general disorder such as pseudo-elastic xanthoma, Ehles Danlos syndrome, Paget's disease and hemoglobinopathies. It is a pathology that generally remains asymptomatic and would be discovered fortuitously during an ophthalmological examination. Clinical signs such as reduced visual acuity or macular syndrome are seen when the striae progress towards the macula, or when there is a neovascular complication. The diagnosis of angioid striae is essentially clinical. Additional examinations are recommended if neovascular complications are suspected. OCTA offers a new approach to the study of angioid striae. In the absence of neovascular complications, OCTA can show widening of the foveal vascular circle in the presence of a juxta foveal stria, and capillary rarefaction in the stria area(185).OCTA makes a major contribution to the detection of neovascular complications. In terms of AS, VDNs are predominantly type 2, but manual segmentation can detect the presence of occult NVC at the level of the choriocapillaris or the presence of a fibro-vascular network at the level of Bruch's membrane cracks, which could correspond to the birthplace of an NVC (186,187).

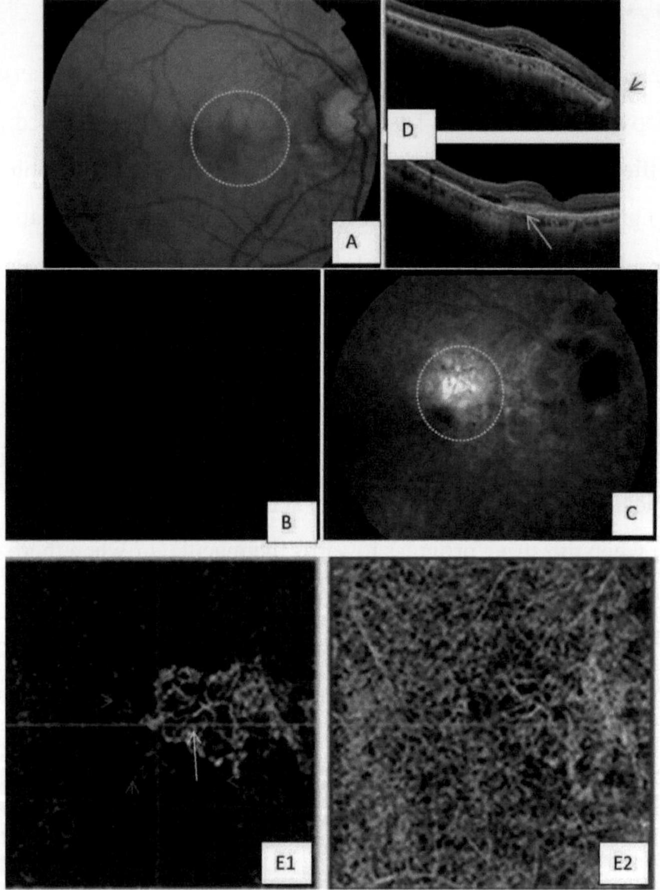

Figure 66: OCTA AND NVC complicating angioid striae.

A 45-year-old man.FO: angioid striae (red arrows) with a greyish-yellow appearance of the macula with a DSR (yellow circle).

Auto-fluorescence image: the striae appear as irregular black lines with a granular appearance all around and inter papillomacular (yellow arrows) (B). AF: inhomogeneous hyper-fluorescence of angioid striae with peri-macular diffusion suggesting the presence of neovascular complication(C). OCT SD(D): Focal ruptures of Bruch's membrane(red arrow) with non-homogeneous DSR content and hyper-reflective fusiform thickening related to a type 2 neo-vessel(yellow arrow).OCTA:Neo-vascular arborization in the outer retina(E1) with peripheral loops (red arrowheads), a central feeder vessel (yellow arrow) and a peri-lesional hypo-signal halo allowing assessment of the activity of this visible type 2 neo-vessel. In the choriocapillaris: visualization of dilated peripheral vessels with decreased vascular density all around (E2).

OCTA offers a risk-free tool for monitoring choroidal neovessels and evaluating response to treatment with intravitreal anti-VEGF injections, while monitoring their size, arrangement, appearance and vascular density. OCTA can be used to estimate NVC activity, but this estimate must remain comparative with other techniques(187).

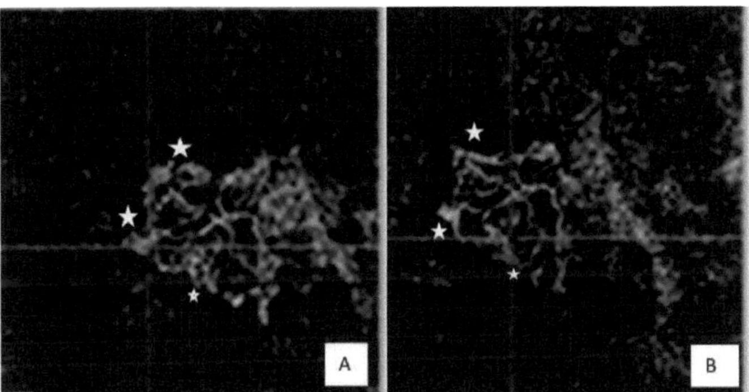

Figure 67: Post-VEGF therapy appearance of NVC complicating angioid streaks by 6*6 mm OCTA slices:
A: initial appearance of CVN /B: post-therapeutic appearance of CVN
At 7 days post intravitreal injection of anti-VEGF, we note the regression of the size of the NVC with rarefaction of the peripheral capillaries and regression of their burls and anastomoses (white stars) with preservation of the large trunks.

As an innocuous test, OCTA enables the detection of NVC recurrence after treatment, but the activity of NVC remains to be assessed by comparing the results provided by OCTA with those of AF and OCT SD.

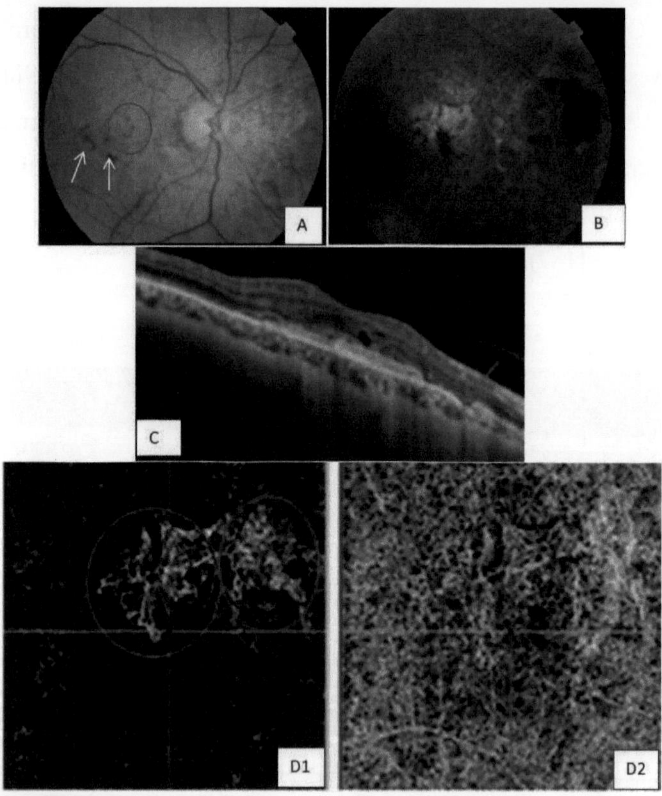

Figure 68: Recurrence of NVC complicating angioid striae :

FO: recurrence of macular haemorrhage in multiple patches (white arrows) temporal to an atropho-pigmentary scar corresponding to the location of the former NVC(red circle)(A).FA (B): non-homogeneous uptake of dye with progressively increasing peri-macular impregnation with late diffusion attenuated by the mask effect secondary to haemorrhage. OCT SD image (C1/C2): diffuse retinal edema with hyper-reflective fusiform thickening over the EP surmounted by cystoid logettes in the outer retina and cracking of Bruch's membrane (blue arrow).OCTA revealed a wheel-spoked neovascular meshwork with a dark peri-lesional halo and multiple anastomotic loops (blue circle) and a central feeder vessel (red arrows).a dead-tree appearance with disorganized capillaries corresponding to the remnant of the initial neovascular network (red circle) objectified in the outer retina(D1) and choriocapillaris(D2).

9.2. OCTA and best's disease :

Vitelliform macular dystrophy or Best's disease is an autosomal dominant disorder of variable expressivity and incomplete penetrance. It is caused by a mutation in the VMD2 gene located on the long arm of chromosome 11, resulting in an accumulation of lipofushin in the form of a characteristic yellow subretinal deposit. Onset is between 7 and 12 years of age, on the occasion of a unilateral or bilateral drop in central visual acuity, metamorphopsia or by chance. The disease passes through various stages in FO: the pre-vitelliform stage, the vitelliform stage, the remodeling stage, the ultimate atrophic stage of the disease with a large patch of centromacular atrophy, and the fibro-glial stage. The diagnosis of Best's disease is essentially clinical.(188) The electro-oculogram makes the diagnosis in doubtful cases, with a typical Arden ratio < 145. Multimodal imaging is used to classify the disease and detect possible complications. In Best's disease, OCTA detects abnormalities in vascular microarchitecture, with a rarefaction of vascular density in the various layers, which is more pronounced in the PVP and choriocapillaris (189). Vascular morphology may be normal in the PVS, but an enlarged ZAC with rupture of the perifoveal anastomotic circle is present in 2/3 of cases, and these anomalies are constant in the PVP(190,191).Signal abnormalities are secondary to the accumulation of lipofushin, giving a non-vascular decorrelation hyper-signal with hypo-signal lesions visible above all in the chorio-capillary zone in the form of a peripheral peri-lesional halo present in 90 Z of cases, which could be due to vascular repression by the vitelline deposits, where blood flow would be weakened and below the detection threshold (191).

OCTA performed in the majority of eyes with vitelliform deposits was subject to some degree of automatic segmentation failure, particularly when the sub-retinal deposits distorted the local anatomy giving rise to projection artefacts with interpretation errors.It is thus sometimes necessary to resort to manual segmentation following the lesional boundaries(191,192).

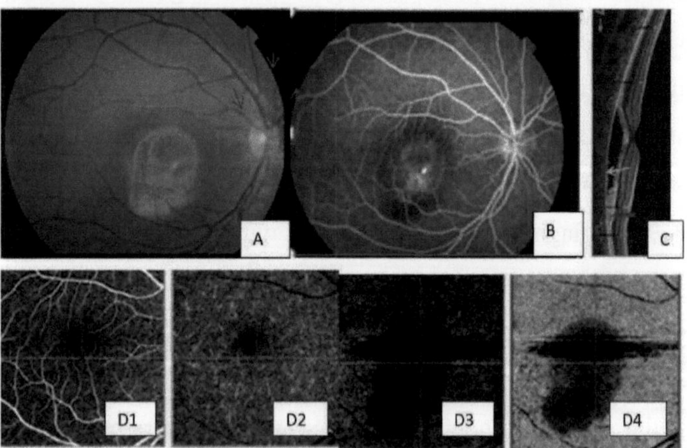

Figure 69: OCTA and BEST disease in the vitelliform stage.

FO(A): a yellowish egg-yolk deposit spread in a dish in a 7-year-old girl.AF(B): the central disc is visible with peripheral inhomogeneous hyper fluorescence due to alteration of the pigment epithelium with central hypo fluorescence due to mask effect secondary to vitelliform deposits. OCT SD of(C) OD shows domed uplift of all retinal layers with DSR and granular hyperreflective appearance of the PE (blue arrow) with hyperreflective splitting of the outer layers by vitelliform material deposition (green arrow).OCTA image: normal PVS (D1), perifoveal capillary rarefaction (red arrows) with widening of the ZAC and capillary dilatation localized to the PVP (D2); in the outer retina and capillary chorio (D3/D4), areas of a signal secondary to the absence of decorrelation by masking due to DSR and vitelliform material.

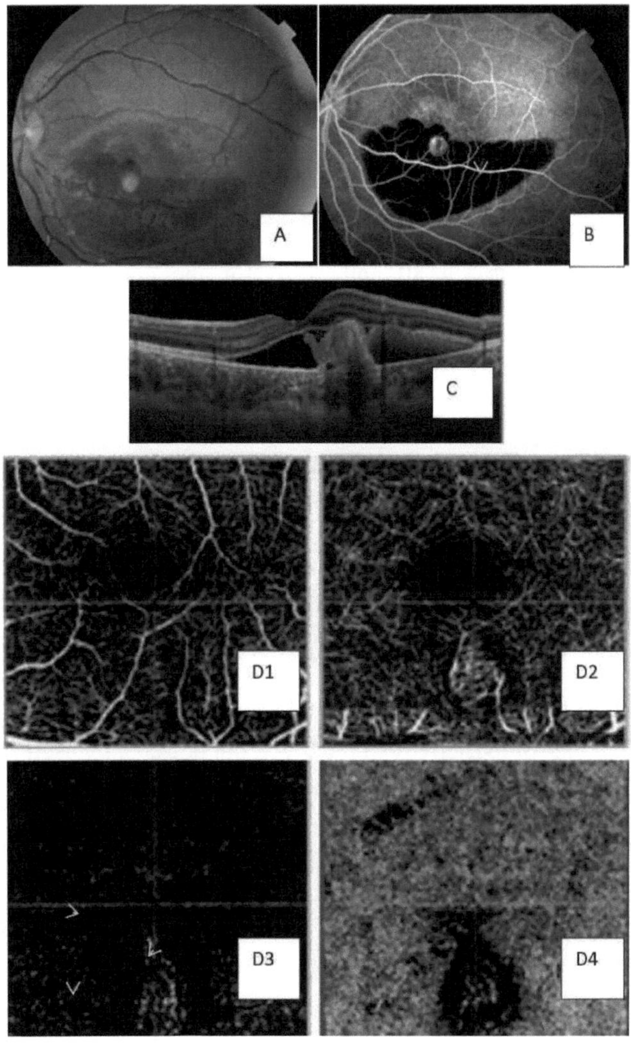

Figure 70: CVN complicating BEST disease :
7-year-old girl: FO(A): presence of central yellowish material with inferior sub-retinal hemorrhage(A). FA(B): inhomogeneous uptake of fluo at the level of the central lesion with progressive impregnation and diffusion suggesting the presence of active choroidal neovascularization. OCT(C) shows a retinal uplift with hyper-reflective content corresponding to sub-retinal haemorrhage and sub-retinal deposits with posterior shadow cone, and at the level of which we note a discontinuity in the EP).
OCTA image: normal-looking PVS(D1),decreased vascular density in the deep plexus with rarefaction of the perifoveal anastomotic circle and localized capillary dilatation(D2).in the outer retina(D3) and the Choriocapillaris (D4), we note the presence of a neovascular network in the form of glomeruli(arrowheads)with evidence of the feeder vessel .

OCTA has been shown to be superior to FA for the detection of neovascular complications. Indeed, the sensitivity and specificity of OCTA vary between 80 and 100Z for the detection of NVC according to different studies(193,194). The morphological characteristics of this neo-vessel can be analysed by measuring its size, although this detection may be hampered by masking due to the accumulation of vitelline material, which makes the detection of hyper-fluorescence impossible. This hyper-fluorescence, if present, together with secondary dye leakage, makes analysis of the morphological characteristics of the CVN difficult(193,194). However, FA is still superior to OCTA for assessing the activity of the CVN, and therefore for making therapeutic decisions. OCTA gives an idea of the activity of the CVN, but does not by itself enable a CVN to be treated. OCTA can be used for post-treatment monitoring of CVNs, and to detect quiescent CVNs in the contralateral eye.

9.3. Severe myopia and its neovascular complication:

Severe myopia is a major cause of reduced visual acuity, which has been steadily increasing in recent years. Neovascular complication is a major cause that threatens central vision, with a poor prognosis. The gold standard for the diagnosis of NVC in myopia is FA associated with SD OCT, which shows the presence of hyper-reflective material generally above the EP, with or without the presence of exudative signs. VNM appears on OCTA as a loose lace with filamentous vessels or a tortuous capillary network with numerous vascular branches in heterogeneous hyper signal above the PE in the majority of cases(195-197). The sensitivity of OCTA for the detection of myopic CVN varies from 90.48 Z according to Querques et al (198) to 94.1 Z according to Myata et al, with a specificity of 100 Z(197) . The lack of visualization of the CVN is due to the turbulent flow within the CVN or to the small size of the neovascular membrane. This characteristic makes the CVN appear smaller than that seen on FA, due to the absence of visualization of all the CVN meshes and filaments, in addition to the diffusion of fluorescein on FA(199,200).

To obtain the best view of the vascular network, manual segmentation is used just above the EP band. Pathological myopia is often characterized by posterior macular staphyloma, irregular surface, atrophic EP, choroidal thinning, which make automatic segmentation difficult, giving rise to segmentation artifacts. OCTA in the evaluation of myopic eyes is not a stand-alone imaging test. It is part of a broader multimodal imaging system that can better characterize VDN and aid therapeutic decision-making. In addition,

OCTA has revealed alterations in the retinal microvascular network in very myopic eyes, correlating with lengthening of the axial length and a decrease in vascular density at the PVS and PVP. There is also a decrease in choroidal blood flow due to increased vascular resistance and narrowing of the posterior ciliary artery. Fractal analysis of the micro-vascularization by OCTA images can help characterize the underlying pathophysiological mechanisms involved in myopia(203).

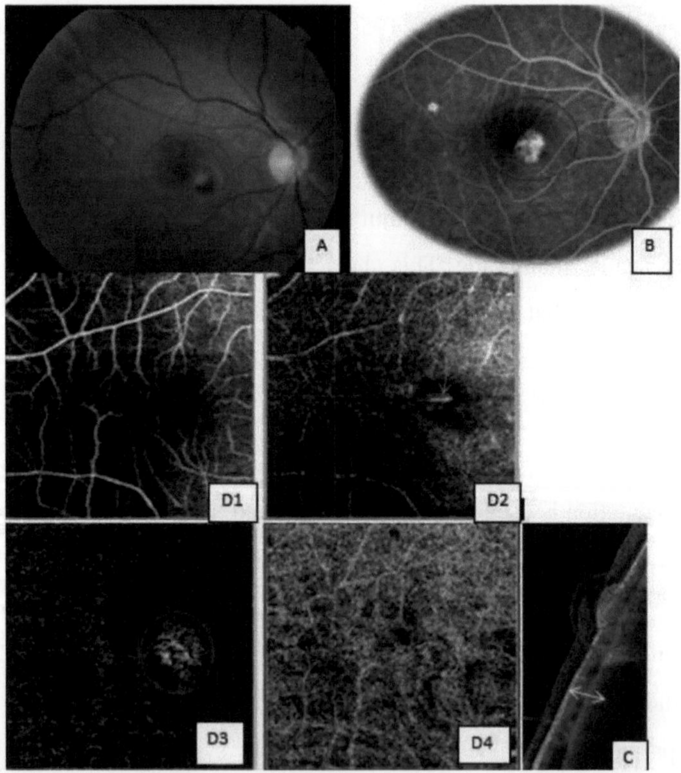

Figure 71: Myopic CVN and OCTA.
A 30-year-old lady with -7.5 dioptres high myopia FO: examination revealed neovascular membrane with peri-macular haemorrhage (red circle)(A).early

hyper-fluorescence FA that increases during the angiographic sequence with DSR. The boundaries of the NVM remain difficult to assess due to dye diffusion(B).SD OCT: fusiform hyper-reflectivity above the PE with thickening of the retinal layers opposite it in favour of an active type 2 CVN. SD OCT shows the presence of retinal atrophy (red arrow) with decreased choroidal thickness (yellow arrow) which are signs in favour of high myopia(C).

OCTA shows conservation of the normal architecture of the PVS(D1)with the presence of an abnormal flow in asignal at the level of the PVP in hyper signal(red arrow) surrounded by a dense halo in hypo signal (blue arrow)(D2).the abnormal arborization appears more identifiable in the outer retina (red circle), which appears dense in hyper signal with wheel-shaped capillaries(D3).in the choriocapillaris, capillary rarefaction is noted with the presence of areas in a signal(D4).

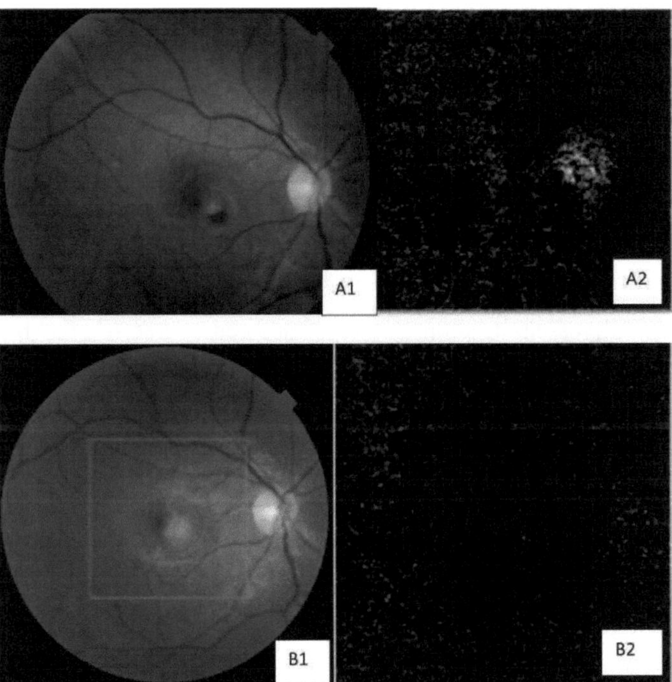

Figure 72: Post-therapy OCTA appearance of myopic CVN.
A1/A2: initial appearance. B1/B2: post-therapy appearance
The patient underwent an intravitreal injection of anti-VEGF, at 15 days post-injection: the haemorrhage disappeared, leaving an atrophic scar (A1/B1). OCTA showed regression in the size of the NVC, with capillary rarefaction giving a dead-tree appearance (A2/B2).

9.4. Idiopathic CVN in young people:

Idiopathic choroidal neovascularization, a unilateral eye disease that occurs in patients under 50 years of age and is diagnosed when the cause of choroidal neovascularization is undetermined, accounts for around 17% of patients with CVN(204). These neovessels are derived from the choroidal vasculature and penetrate through Bruch's membrane into the subretinal space, which is typical of type 2 CVN. Currently, in clinical situations, FA and A ICG are the reference standard for the detection of CVN (204).OCTA has shown superiority for the detection of idiopathic CVN. Indeed, CVN structures were varied, generally irregular or almost round, with internal arborescent capillaries. They appeared as irregular, tightly bound outflow formations in the outer retinal layer. Most of the abnormal vessels in idiopathic CVN showed a "tree-in-bud" blood flow which suggested that idiopathic CVN are composed of numerous tightly coiled blood vessels, in which blood flowing through several turns or knotted parts is likely to form turbulence making detection of individual neovascular loops difficult as OCTA only measures linear blood flow(205,206). The turbulent movement then appears as a dark area.

OCTA also demonstrated peripheral blood flow around the VNM. It has been suggested that these lesions may have an anastomotic vessel delineating the outer edge of the vascular lesions, which have played an important role in the pathophysiology of CVN(204).

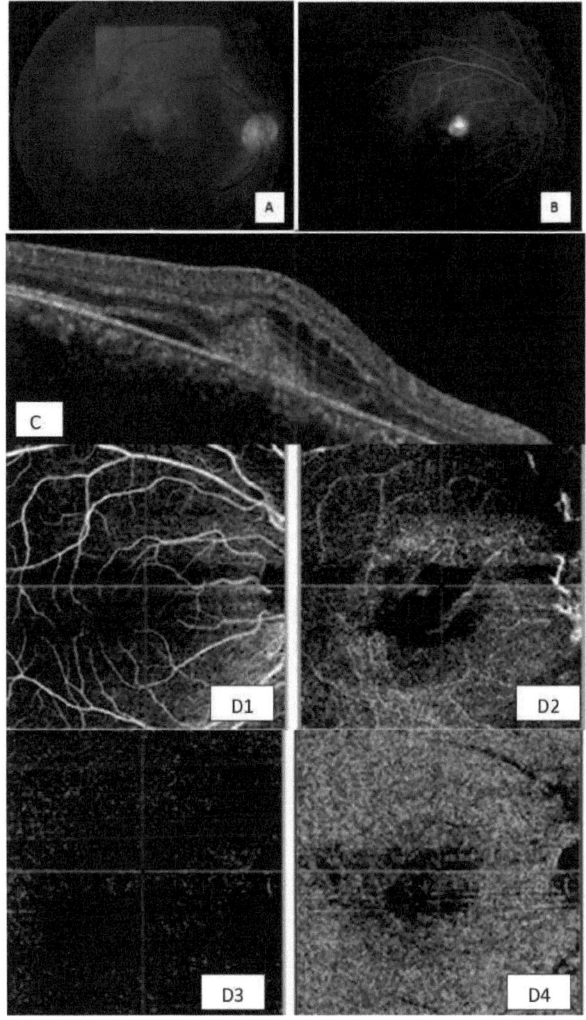

Figure 73: Idiopathic CVN in young subjects.
16-year-old girl with no notable history, emmetropic. FO (A): yellowish macular thickening with deep hemorrhage in favor of NVC.AF(B): macular hyperfluorescence with diffusion. OCT B scan(C): presence of a hyper-reflective thickening above the EP with the presence of a hyper-reflective intraretinal hemorrhage. We also note the presence of a multi-lobular DSR with cystoid OM, in favor of an active type 2 CVN. On OCTA, the perifoveal anastomotic circle is broken at the PVS(D1). The appearance of the ZAC was difficult to assess in the PVP (D2) due to masking by the haemorrhage

and the DSR. A hyper-dense abnormal signal could be identified in the outer retina (D3), although its characteristics could not be identified, but its size appeared to be smaller than that of the FA. Manual segmentation would have enabled a better analysis of the characteristics of the MNV.

10. CONCLUSION

OCTA is a new imaging technique that has revolutionized the exploration and understanding of the pathophysiology of non-inflammatory chorio-retinal pathologies. This technique enables visualization of the microcirculation with high depth resolution, in the absence of image masking by dye leakage or diffusion, giving images with good contrast. In fact, volumetric data can be segmented and OCTA from different retinal layers can be projected to allow separate visualization of retinal plexi-capillaries and chorio-capillaries. In addition, OCTA images can be viewed in cross-section to confirm the deep location of vascular pathology, as structural OCT data are acquired simultaneously with OCTA data and it is therefore possible to display both en face and cross-sectional structural OCT images that are intrinsically co-registered with OCTA data.

OCTA is an innocuous examination that requires no injection of dye, and can be repeated. It has become an important tool for studying and monitoring various non-inflammatory chorio-retinal pathologies. In AMD, OCTA has made it possible to modify the nomenclature of choroidal neovessels, while clarifying their relationship with retinal PE without the need for FA. The detection of choroidal neovascularization is a major contribution of OCTA in monitoring patients with chronic CRSC. For the study of diabetic maculopathy, although structural OCT enables analysis of DME, OCTA has enabled better study of ischemic maculopathy, while allowing separate visualization of PVS and PVP, whose level of damage is proportional to peripheral retinal ischemia. In the case of venous occlusions, OCTA has made it possible to quantify the degree of initial damage and to assess the presence of reperfusion networks, enabling visual prognosis to be estimated. OCTA has also enabled us to gain a better understanding of myopic maculopathy, and to detect neovascular complications.

Like any new imaging technique, OCTA has certain limitations: on the one hand, imaging protocols require the same retinal position to be re-analyzed several times. As a result, OCTA requires higher imaging speeds or longer imaging times than structural OCT, making it sensitive to various sources of artifact. OCTA images can present far more artifacts than structural images, with the risk of misinterpretation, since a decorrelation signal can be obtained even in the absence of movement, as in hard exudates or certain small hemorrhages, and the smallest vessels with very low flow may not cause a decorrelation signal, and therefore be invisible.

On the other hand, OCTA, being a static test, cannot assess alterations in vascular permeability or leakage, which are usually visualized using AF or ICGA. In addition, the appearance of OCTA image data is highly dependent on the details of the OCT instrument, scanning protocols, signal processing and the methods used to generate OCTA information from structural OCT data.

11. BIBLIOGRAPHY

1. Gao SS, Jia Y, Zhang M, Su JP, Liu G, Hwang TS, et al. Optical Coherence Tomography Angiography. Investigative Ophthalmology & Visual Science. 13 Jul 2016;57(9):OCT27.

2. Spaide RF, Fujimoto JG, Waheed NK, Sadda SR, Staurenghi G. Optical coherence tomography angiography. Progress in Retinal and Eye Research [Internet]. dec 2017 [cited 2018 March 17]; Available from: http://linkinghub.elsevier.com/retrieve/pii/S1350946217300563

3. Jia Y, Tan O, Tokayer J, Potsaid B, Wang Y, Liu JJ, et al. Split-spectrum amplitudedecorrelation angiography with optical coherence tomography. Opt Express. Feb 13, 2012;20(4):4710-25.

4. Khadamy J. Optical Coherence Tomography Angiography (OCTA) in Ophthalmology; Technology, Pros, Cons and Commercial Prototypes. JOJ Ophthalmology [Internet]. Apr 19, 2017 [cited 2018 March 17];2(5). Available from: https://juniperpublishers.com/jojo/JOJO.MS.ID.555598.php

5. Kashani AH, Chen C-L, Gahm JK, Zheng F, Richter GM, Rosenfeld PJ, et al. Optical coherence tomography angiography: A comprehensive review of current methods and clinical applications. Progress in Retinal and Eye Research. sept 2017;60:66-100.

6. de Carlo TE, Romano A, Waheed NK, Duker JS. A review of optical coherence tomography angiography (OCTA). International Journal of Retina and Vitreous [Internet]. apr 2015 [cited 2018 March 17];1(1). Available from: http://journalretinavitreous.biomedcentral.com/articles/10.1186/s40942-015-0005- 8

7. Sambhav K, Grover S, Chalam KV. The application of optical coherence tomography angiography in retinal diseases. Survey of Ophthalmology. nov 2017;62(6):838-66.

8. Wylçgala A, Teper S, Dobrowolski D, Wylçgala E. Optical coherence angiography: A review. Medicine. oct 2016;95(41):e4907.

9. Tan ACS, Tan GS, Denniston AK, Keane PA, Ang M, Milea D, et al. An overview of the clinical applications of optical coherence tomography angiography. Eye (Lond). Feb 2018;32(2):262-86.

10. Gorczynska I, Migacz JV, Zawadzki RJ, Capps AG, Werner JS. Comparison of amplitude-decorrelation, speckle-variance and phase-

variance OCT angiography methods for imaging the human retina and choroid. Biomed Opt Express. Feb 19, 2016;7(3):911-42.

11. Aumann S, Donner S, Fischer J, Müller F. Optical Coherence Tomography (OCT): Principle and Technical Realization. In: Bille JF, editor. High Resolution Imaging in Microscopy and Ophthalmology: New Frontiers in Biomedical Optics [Internet]. Cham (CH): Springer; 2019 [cited 2020 Mar 22]. Available from: http://www.ncbi.nlm.nih.gov/books/NBK554044/

12. De Oliveira PRC, Berger AR, Chow DR. Optical coherence tomography angiography in chorioretinal disorders. Canadian Journal of Ophthalmology / Journal Canadien d'Ophtalmologie. feb 2017;52(1):125-36.

13. Enders C, Lang GE, Dreyhaupt J, Loidl M, Lang GK, Werner JU. Quantity and quality of image artifacts in optical coherence tomography angiography. PLoS One [Internet]. 25 Jan. 2019 [cited 15 Apr. 2019];14(1). Available from: https://www.ncbi.nlm.nih.gov/pmc/articles/PMC6347178/

14. Spaide RF, Fujimoto JG, Waheed NK. Image artifacts in Optical Coherence Angiography. Retina. nov 2015;35(11):2163-80.

15. Ang M, Tan ACS, Cheung CMG, Keane PA, Dolz-Marco R, Sng CCA, et al. Optical coherence tomography angiography: a review of current and future clinical applications. Graefe's Archive for Clinical and Experimental Ophthalmology. feb 2018;256(2):237-45.

16. Lozzi A, Agrawal A, Boretsky A, Welle CG, Hammer DX. Image quality metrics for optical coherence angiography. Biomed Opt Express. June 12, 2015;6(7):2435-47.

17. Bandello F, Corbelli E, Carnevali A, Pierro L, Querques G. Optical Coherence Tomography Angiography of Diabetic Retinopathy. In: Bandello F, Souied EH, Querques G, editors. Developments in Ophthalmology [Internet]. S. Karger AG; 2016 [cited 2018 Mar 20]. p. 107-12. Available from: https://www.karger.com/ Article/FullText/442801

18. Chung CY, Tang HHY, Li SH, Li KKW. Differential microvascular assessment of retinal vein occlusion with coherence tomography angiography and fluorescein angiography: a blinded comparative study. International Ophthalmology [Internet]. 26 May 2017 [cited 17 March 2018]; Available from: http://link.springer.com/10.1007/s10792-017-0570-y

19. Kim K, Kim ES, Yu S-Y. Optical coherence tomography angiography

analysis of foveal microvascular changes and inner retinal layer thinning in patients with diabetes. British Journal of Ophthalmology. Dec 19, 2017;bjophthalmol-2017- 311149.

20. Veritti D, Sarao V, Francescutti L, Rota N, Loewenstein A, Borrelli E, et al. Optical coherence tomography angiography findings in diabetic retinopathy. Expert Review of Ophthalmology. 2 Nov 2017;12(6):475-84.

21. Mendis KR, Balaratnasingam C, Yu P, Barry CJ, McAllister IL, Cringle SJ, et al. Correlation of histologic and clinical images to determine the diagnostic value of fluorescein angiography for studying retinal capillary detail. Invest Ophthalmol Vis Sci. Nov 2010;51(11):5864-9.

22. Matsunaga DR, Yi JJ, De Koo LO, Ameri H, Puliafito CA, Kashani AH. Optical Coherence Tomography Angiography of Diabetic Retinopathy in Human Subjects. Ophthalmic Surgery, Lasers and Imaging Retina. 1 Sep 2015;46(8):796-805.

23. Hasegawa N, Nozaki M, Takase N, Yoshida M, Ogura Y. New Insights Into Microaneurysms in the Deep Capillary Plexus Detected by Optical Coherence Tomography Angiography in Diabetic Macular Edema. Invest Ophthalmol Vis Sci. 01 2016;57(9):OCT348-355.

24. Horii T, Murakami T, Nishijima K, Sakamoto A, Ota M, Yoshimura N. Optical Coherence Tomographic Characteristics of Microaneurysms in Diabetic Retinopathy. American Journal of Ophthalmology. dec 2010;150(6):840-848.e1.

25. Couturier A, Mané V, Bonnin S, Erginay A, Massin P, Gaudric A, et al. CAPILLARY PLEXUS ANOMALIES IN DIABETIC RETINOPATHY ON OPTICAL COHERENCE TOMOGRAPHY ANGIOGRAPHY: Retina. nov 2015;35(11):2384-91.

26. Parravano M, De Geronimo D, Scarinci F, Querques L, Virgili G, Simonett JM, et al. Diabetic Microaneurysms Internal Reflectivity on Spectral-Domain Optical Coherence Tomography and Optical Coherence Tomography Angiography Detection. American Journal of Ophthalmology. july 2017;179:90-6.

27. Hwang TS, Gao SS, Liu L, Lauer AK, Bailey ST, Flaxel CJ, et al. Automated
Quantification of Capillary Nonperfusion Using Optical Coherence Tomography Angiography in Diabetic Retinopathy. JAMA Ophthalmol. 1 Apr.
2016;134(4):367-73.

28. Khadamy J, Abri Aghdam K, Falavarjani KG. An Update on Optical

Coherence Tomography Angiography in Diabetic Retinopathy. J Ophthalmic Vis Res. 2018;13(4):487-97.

29. Sandhu HS, Eladawi N, Elmogy M, Keynton R, Helmy O, Schaal S, et al. Automated diabetic retinopathy detection using optical coherence tomography angiography: a pilot study. British Journal of Ophthalmology. 23 Jan 2018;bjophthalmol-2017-311489.

30. Russell JF, Flynn HW, Sridhar J, Townsend JH, Shi Y, Fan KC, et al. Distribution of Diabetic Neovascularization on Ultra-Widefield Fluorescein Angiography and on Simulated Widefield OCT Angiography. American Journal of Ophthalmology. nov 2019;207:110-20.

31. Nesper PL, Soetikno BT, Zhang HF, Fawzi AA. OCT angiography and visible-light OCT in diabetic retinopathy. Vision Research. oct 2017;139:191-203.

32. Pan J, Chen D, Yang X, Zou R, Zhao K, Cheng D, et al. Characteristics of Neovascularization in Early Stages of Proliferative Diabetic Retinopathy by Optical Coherence Tomography Angiography. Am J Ophthalmol. 2018;192:146-56.

33. Ishibazawa A, Nagaoka T, Yokota H, Takahashi A, Omae T, Song Y-S, et al. Characteristics of Retinal Neovascularization in Proliferative Diabetic Retinopathy Imaged by Optical Coherence Tomography Angiography. Invest Ophthalmol Vis Sci. 01 2016;57(14):6247-55.

34. Spaide RF, Klancnik JM, Cooney MJ. Retinal Vascular Layers Imaged by Fluorescein Angiography and Optical Coherence Tomography Angiography. JAMA Ophthalmology. Jan 1, 2015;133(1):45.

35. Barthelmes D, Sutter FKP, Gillies MC. Differential optical densities of intraretinal spaces. Investigative Ophthalmology and Visual Science. 2008;49(8):3529-34.

36. Spaide RF. Volume-Rendered Optical Coherence Tomography of Diabetic Retinopathy Pilot Study. American Journal of Ophthalmology. Dec 1, 2015;160(6):1200-10.

37. Sorour OA, Sabrosa AS, Yasin Alibhai A, Arya M, Ishibazawa A, Witkin AJ, et al. Optical coherence tomography angiography analysis of macular vessel density before and after anti-VEGF therapy in eyes with diabetic retinopathy. Int Ophthalmol. 1 Oct 2019;39(10):2361-71.

38. CORRELATION BETWEEN CYSTOID SPACES IN CHRONIC DIABETIC MACULAR EDEMA AND CAPILLARY NONPERFUSION DETECTED BY OPTICAL COHERENCE TOMOGRAPHY

ANGIOGRAPHY [Internet]. [cited 16 Dec 2019]. Available from: https://insights.ovid.com/article/00006982-201612001- 00011

39. Onishi AC, Nesper PL, Roberts PK, Moharram GA, Chai H, Liu L, et al. Importance of Considering the Middle Capillary Plexus on OCT Angiography in Diabetic Retinopathy. Invest Ophthalmol Vis Sci. 01 2018;59(5):2167-76.

40. Samara WA, Shahlaee A, Adam MK, Khan MA, Chiang A, Maguire JI, et al. Quantification of Diabetic Macular Ischemia Using Optical Coherence Tomography Angiography and Its Relationship with Visual Acuity. Ophthalmology. feb 2017;124(2):235-44.

41. Dupas B, Minvielle W, Bonnin S, Couturier A, Erginay A, Massin P, et al. Association Between Vessel Density and Visual Acuity in Patients With Diabetic Retinopathy and Poorly Controlled Type 1 Diabetes. JAMA Ophthalmol. 01 2018;136(7):721-8.

42. de Carlo TE, Chin AT, Joseph T, Baumal CR, Witkin AJ, Duker JS, et al. Distinguishing Diabetic Macular Edema From Capillary Nonperfusion Using Optical Coherence Tomography Angiography. Ophthalmic Surg Lasers Imaging Retina. feb 2016;47(2):108-14.

43. Bonnin S, Mané V, Couturier A, Julien M, Paques M, Tadayoni R, et al. NEW INSIGHT INTO THE MACULAR DEEP VASCULAR PLEXUS IMAGED BY OPTICAL COHERENCE TOMOGRAPHY ANGIOGRAPHY: Retina. nov 2015;35(11):2347-52.

44. Cao J, McLeod DS, Merges CA, Lutty GA. Choriocapillaris Degeneration and Related Pathologic Changes in Human Diabetic Eyes. Arch Ophthalmol. May 1, 1998;116(5):589-97.

45. Shiragami C, Shiraga F, Matsuo T, Tsuchida Y, Ohtsuki H. Risk factors for diabetic choroidopathy in patients with diabetic retinopathy. Graefes Arch Clin Exp Ophthalmol. June 2002;240(6):436-42.

46. Endo H, Kase S, Takahashi M, Yokoi M, Isozaki C, Katsuta S, et al. Alteration of layer thickness in the choroid of diabetic patients. Clinical & Experimental Ophthalmology [Internet]. [cited 11 Jan 2020];n/a(n/a). Available from: https://onlinelibrary.wiley.com/doi/abs/10.1111/ceo.13199

47. Wang JC, Laíns I, Providência J, Armstrong GW, Santos AR, Gil P, et al. Diabetic Choroidopathy: Choroidal Vascular Density and Volume in Diabetic Retinopathy With Swept-Source Optical Coherence Tomography. American Journal of Ophthalmology. Dec 1, 2017;184:75-83.

48. Ferrara D, Waheed NK, Duker JS. Investigating the choriocapillaris and choroidal vasculature with new optical coherence tomography technologies. Progress in Retinal and Eye Research. May 1, 2016;52:130-55.

49. Conti FF, Qin VL, Rodrigues EB, Sharma S, Rachitskaya AV, Ehlers JP, et al. Choriocapillaris and retinal vascular plexus density of diabetic eyes using splitspectrum amplitude decorrelation spectral-domain optical coherence tomography angiography. British Journal of Ophthalmology. Apr 1, 2019;103(4):452-6.

50. Yang J, Wang E, Zhao X, Xia S, Yuan M, Chen H, et al. Optical coherence tomography angiography analysis of the choriocapillary layer in treatment-naïve diabetic eyes. Graefes Arch Clin Exp Ophthalmol. july 2019;257(7):1393-9.

51. Keane PA, Patel PJ, Liakopoulos S, Heussen FM, Sadda SR, Tufail A. Evaluation of Age-related Macular Degeneration With Optical Coherence Tomography. Survey of Ophthalmology. Sep 1, 2012;57(5):389-414.

52. Ma J, Desai R, Nesper P, Gill M, Fawzi A, Skondra D. Optical Coherence Tomographic Angiography Imaging in Age-Related Macular Degeneration. Ophthalmology and Eye Diseases. jan 2017;9:117917211668607.

53. Haouchine B, Gaudric A. OCT in age-related macular degeneration /data/revues/01815512/00300HS1/56/ [Internet]. 2008 Mar 8 [cited 2019 Dec 24]; Available from: https://www.em-consulte.com/en/article/113514

54. Srour M, Semoun O, Miere A, Souied E. Will OCT-angiography revolutionize AMD imaging practice? 2016;4.

55. Alten F, Lauermann JL, Clemens CR, Heiduschka P, Eter N. Signal reduction in choriocapillaris and segmentation errors in spectral domain OCT angiography caused by soft drusen. Graefes Arch Clin Exp Ophthalmol. 1 Dec 2017;255(12):2347-55.

56. Querques G, Miere A, Souied EH. Optical Coherence Tomography Angiography Features of Type 3 Neovascularization in Age-Related Macular Degeneration. In: Bandello F, Souied EH, Querques G, editors. Developments in Ophthalmology [Internet]. S. Karger AG; 2016 [cited 23 Apr 2019]. p. 57-61. Available from: https://www.karger.com/Article/FullText/442779

57. NESPER PL, SOETIKNO BT, FAWZI AA. Choriocapillaris Non-Perfusion is Associated with Poor Visual Acuity in Eyes with Reticular Pseudodrusen. Am J Ophthalmol. Feb 2017;174:42-55.

58. Alten F, Heiduschka P, Clemens CR, Eter N. Exploring Choriocapillaris under reticular pseudodrusen using OCT-Angiography. Graefes Arch Clin Exp Ophthalmol. 1 Nov 2016;254(11):2165-73.

59. Querques G, Souied EH. Vascularized Drusen: Slowly Progressive Type 1 Neovascularization Mimicking Drusenoid Retinal Pigment Epithelium Elevation. RETINA. dec 2015;35(12):2433-2439.

60. Or C, Heier JS, Boyer D, Brown D, Shah S, Alibhai AY, et al. Vascularized drusen: a cross-sectional study. Int J Retina Vitreous [Internet]. 20 Aug. 2019 [cited 24 Dec. 2019];5. Available from: https://www.ncbi.nlm.nih.gov/pmc/articles/PMC6702713/

61. Chatziralli I, Theodossiadis G, Panagiotidis D, Pousoulidi P, Theodossiadis P. Choriocapillaris Vascular Density Changes in Patients with Drusen: Cross-Sectional Study Based on Optical Coherence Tomography Angiography Findings. Ophthalmology and Therapy. June 2018;7(1):101 -7.

62. Iafe NA, Phasukkijwatana N, Chen X, Sarraf D. Retinal Capillary Density and Foveal Avascular Zone Area Are Age-Dependent: Quantitative Analysis Using Optical Coherence Tomography Angiography. Investigative Ophthalmology & Visual Science. 28 Oct 2016;57(13):5780.

63. Lauermann JL, Eter N, Alten F. Optical Coherence Tomography Angiography Offers New Insights into Choriocapillaris Perfusion. Ophthalmologica. 2018;239(2-3):74-84.

64. Roisman L, Goldhardt R. OCT Angiography: an Upcoming Non-invasive Tool for Diagnosis of Age-Related Macular Degeneration. Current Ophthalmology Reports. June 2017;5(2):136-40.

65. Schneider EW, Fowler SC. Optical coherence tomography angiography in the management of age-related macular degeneration: Current Opinion in Ophthalmology. may 2018;29(3):217-25.

66. Grossniklaus HE, Green WR. Choroidal neovascularization. American Journal of Ophthalmology. March 1, 2004;137(3):496-503.

67. Green WR, Enger C. Age-related Macular Degeneration Histopathologic Studies: The 1992 Lorenz E. Zimmerman Lecture. Ophthalmology. 1993 Oct 1;100(10):1519-35.

68. Schmidt-Erfurth U, Waldstein SM. A paradigm shift in imaging biomarkers in neovascular age-related macular degeneration. Progress in Retinal and Eye Research. 1 Jan 2016;50:1-24.

69. Castillo MM, Mowatt G, Elders A, Lois N, Fraser C, Hernández R, et al.

Optical Coherence Tomography for the Monitoring of Neovascular Age-Related Macular Degeneration: A Systematic Review. Ophthalmology. Feb 1, 2015;122(2):399-406.

70. Coscas GJ, Lupidi M, Coscas F, Cagini C, Souied EH. OPTICAL COHERENCE TOMOGRAPHY ANGIOGRAPHY VERSUS TRADITIONAL MULTIMODAL IMAGING IN ASSESSING THE ACTIVITY OF EXUDATIVE AGE-RELATED MACULAR DEGENERATION: A New Diagnostic Challenge. Retina. nov 2015;35(11):2219-28.

71. Ahmed D, Stattin M, Graf A, Forster J, Glittenberg C, Krebs I, et al. DETECTION OF TREATMENT-NAIVE CHOROIDAL NEOVASCULARIZATION IN AGE- RELATED MACULAR DEGENERATION BY SWEPT SOURCE OPTICAL COHERENCE TOMOGRAPHY ANGIOGRAPHY: Retina. nov 2018;38(11):2143-9.

72. Bailey ST, Thaware O, Wang J, Hagag AM, Zhang X, Flaxel CJ, et al. Detection of Nonexudative Choroidal Neovascularization and Progression to Exudative Choroidal Neovascularization Using OCT Angiography. Ophthalmology Retina. August 2019;3(8):629-36.

73. Liang M, Carlo T de, Baumal C, Reichel E, Waheed N, Duker J, et al. CORRELATION OF SPECTRAL DOMAIN OPTICAL COHERENCE TOMOGRAPHY ANGIOGRAPHY AND CLINICAL ACTIVITY IN NEOVASCULAR AGE-RELATED MACULAR DEGENERATION. Retina. dec 2016;36(12):2265-73.

74. Lumbroso B, Rispoli M, Savastano MC, Jia Y, Tan O, Huang D. Optical Coherence Tomography Angiography Study of Choroidal Neovascularization Early Response after Treatment. Dev Ophthalmol. 2016;56:77-85.

75. Al-Sheikh M, Iafe NA, Phasukkijwatana N, Sadda SR, Sarraf D. Biomarkers of Neovascular Activity in Age-Related Macular Degeneration Using Oct Angiography. Retina. 2018;38(2):220-30.

76. Coscas F, Lupidi M, Boulet JF, Sellam A, Cabral D, Serra R, et al. Optical coherence tomography angiography in exudative age-related macular degeneration: a predictive model for treatment decisions. British Journal of Ophthalmology. 22 Nov 2018;bjophthalmol-2018-313065.

77. Coscas G, Lupidi M, Coscas F, Français C, Cagini C, Souied EH. Optical Coherence Tomography Angiography during Follow-Up: Qualitative and Quantitative Analysis of Mixed Type I and II Choroidal Neovascularization after Vascular Endothelial Growth Factor Trap Therapy. Ophthalmic Research. 2015;54(2):57-63.

78. Carnevali A, Cicinelli MV, Capuano V, Corvi F, Mazzaferro A, Querques L, et al. Optical Coherence Tomography Angiography: A Useful Tool for Diagnosis of Treatment-Naive Quiescent Choroidal Neovascularization. American Journal of Ophthalmology. Sep 1, 2016;169:189-98.

79. Inoue M, Jung JJ, Balaratnasingam C, Dansingani KK, Dhrami-Gavazi E, Suzuki M, et al. A Comparison Between Optical Coherence Tomography Angiography and Fluorescein Angiography for the Imaging of Type 1 Neovascularization. Invest Ophthalmol Vis Sci. 1 Jul 2016;57(9):OCT314-23.

80. Sulzbacher F, Pollreisz A, Kaider A, Kickinger S, Sacu S, Schmidt-Erfurth U. Identification and clinical role of choroidal neovascularization characteristics based on optical coherence tomography angiography. Acta Ophthalmologica. 2017;95(4):414-20.

81. Kuehlewein L, Bansal M, Lenis TL, Iafe NA, Sadda SR, Filho MAB, et al. Optical Coherence Tomography Angiography of Type 1 Neovascularization in Age-Related Macular Degeneration. American Journal of Ophthalmology. Oct 1, 2015;160(4):739-748.e2.

82. Xu D, Dávila JP, Rahimi M, Rebhun CB, Alibhai AY, Waheed NK, et al. Longterm Progression of Type 1 Neovascularization in Age-related Macular Degeneration Using Optical Coherence Tomography Angiography. American Journal of Ophthalmology. march 2018;187:10-20.

83. Farecki M-L, Gutfleisch M, Faatz H, Rothaus K, Heimes B, Spital G, et al. Characteristics of type 1 and 2 CNV in exudative AMD in OCT-Angiography. Graefes Arch Clin Exp Ophthalmol. May 1, 2017;255(5):913-21.

84. A EA, Sy C, O S, A M, M S, M Q-EM, et al. TYPE 2 NEOVASCULARIZATION SECONDARY TO AGE-RELATED MACULAR DEGENERATION IMAGED BY OPTICAL COHERENCE TOMOGRAPHY ANGIOGRAPHY. Retina. 1 Nov 2015;35(11):2212-8.

85. Querques G, Atmani K, Berboucha E, Martinelli D, Coscas G, Soubrane G, et al. Angiographic analysis of retinal-choroidal anastomosis by confocal scanning laser ophthalmoscopy technology and corresponding (eye-tracked) spectral-domain optical coherence tomography. Retina (Philadelphia, Pa). Feb 2010;30(2):222-34.

86. Miere A, Querques G, Semoun O, Ameen AE, Capuano V, Souied E. OPTICAL COHERENCE TOMOGRAPHY ANGIOGRAPHY IN EARLY TYPE 3 NEOVASCULARIZATION. Retina. nov 2015;35(11):2236-41.

87. Tan ACS, Dansingani KK, Yannuzzi LA, Sarraf D, Freund KB. TYPE 3 NEOVASCULARIZATION IMAGED WITH CROSS-SECTIONAL AND EN FACE OPTICAL COHERENCE TOMOGRAPHY ANGIOGRAPHY. Retina (Philadelphia, Pa). feb 2017;37(2):234-46.

88. Cohen SY, Mrejen S. Imaging of Exudative Age-Related Macular Degeneration: Toward a Shift in the Diagnostic Paradigm? Retina (Philadelphia, Pa). 2017;37(9):1625-9.

89. Muakkassa NW, Chin AT, de Carlo T, Klein KA, Baumal CR, Witkin AJ, et al. CHARACTERIZING THE EFFECT OF ANTI-VASCULAR ENDOTHELIAL GROWTH FACTOR THERAPY ON TREATMENT-NAIVE CHOROIDAL NEOVASCULARIZATION USING OPTICAL COHERENCE TOMOGRAPHY ANGIOGRAPHY: Retina. nov 2015;35(11):2252-9.

90. Huang D, Jia Y, Rispoli M, Tan O, Lumbroso B. OCT Angiography of Time Course of Choroidal Neovascularization in Response to Anti-angiogenic Treatment. Retina. nov 2015;35(11):2260-4.

91. pubmeddev, RF S. Optical Coherence Tomography Angiography Signs of Vascular Abnormalization With Antiangiogenic Therapy for Choroidal Neovascularization. - PubMed - NCBI [Internet]. [cited 2019 Dec 26]. Available from: https://www.ncbi.nlm.nih.gov/pubmed/25887628

92. Hikichi T, Agarie M. Reduced Vessel Density of the Choriocapillaris during AntiVascular Endothelial Growth Factor Therapy for Neovascular Age-Related Macular Degeneration. Invest Ophthalmol Vis Sci. March 1, 2019;60(4):1088-95.

93. Miere A, Butori P, Cohen SY, Semoun O, Capuano V, Jung C, et al. VASCULAR REMODELING OF CHOROIDAL NEOVASCULARIZATION AFTER ANTIVASCULAR ENDOTHELIAL GROWTH FACTOR THERAPY VISUALIZED ON OPTICAL COHERENCE TOMOGRAPHY ANGIOGRAPHY: Retina. March 2019;39(3):548-57.

94. Miere A, Semoun O, Cohen S, Ameen AE, Srour M, Jung C, et al. OPTICAL COHERENCE TOMOGRAPHY ANGIOGRAPHY FEATURES OF SUBRETINAL FIBROSIS IN AGE-RELATED MACULAR DEGENERATION. Retina. nov 2015;35(11):2275-84.

95. Amoroso F, Miere A, Semoun O, Jung C, Capuano V, Souied EH. Optical coherence tomography angiography reproducibility of lesion size measurements in neovascular age-related macular degeneration (AMD). British Journal of Ophthalmology. June 2018;102(6):821-6.

96. Coscas G, Lupidi M, Cagini C, Coscas F. 'False-friend' images on optical coherence tomography angiography: early choroidal neovascularization or artifact? Acta Ophthalmologica. 2018;96(2):200-2.

97. Mt B, Cw M, Vj S. Investigation of artifacts in retinal and choroidal OCT angiography with a contrast agent. Biomed Opt Express. Feb 6, 2018;9(3):1020-40.

98. Palkar AH, Khetan V. Polypoidal choroidal vasculopathy: An update on current management and review of literature. Taiwan J Ophthalmol. 2019;9(2):72-92.

99. Kim J-B, Nirwan RS, Kuriyan AE. Polypoidal choroidal vasculopathy. Curr Ophthalmol Rep. June 2017;5(2):176-86.

100. Cheung CMG, Lee WK, Koizumi H, Dansingani K, Lai TYY, Freund KB. Pachychoroid disease. Eye (Lond). jan 2019;33(1):14-33.

101. Cheung CMG, Yanagi Y, Akiba M, Tan A, Mathur R, Chan CM, et al. IMPROVED DETECTION AND DIAGNOSIS OF POLYPOIDAL CHOROIDAL VASCULOPATHY USING A COMBINATION OF OPTICAL COHERENCE TOMOGRAPHY AND OPTICAL COHERENCE TOMOGRAPHY ANGIOGRAPHY: Retina. Sept 2019;39(9):1655-63.

102. FRCSC JY MD, and Efrem D Mandelcorn, MD, Specialist R. Pachychoroid Spectrum: A Closer Look [Internet]. [cited 26 Apr 2020]. Available from: http://www.retina-specialist.com/article/pachychoroid-spectrum-a-closer-look

103. Takayama K, Ito Y, Kaneko H, Kataoka K, Sugita T, Maruko R, et al. Comparison of indocyanine green angiography and optical coherence tomographic angiography in polypoidal choroidal vasculopathy. Eye (Lond). jan 2017;31(1):45-52.

104. Tanaka K, Mori R, Kawamura A, Nakashizuka H, Wakatsuki Y, Yuzawa M. Comparison of OCT angiography and indocyanine green angiographic findings with subtypes of polypoidal choroidal vasculopathy. Br J Ophthalmol. Jan 2017;101(1):51-5.

105. Freund KB, Fine HF. Pachychoroid Disease. Ophthalmic Surg Lasers Imaging Retina. May 4, 2020;51(4):206-9.

106. Gallego-Pinazo R, Dolz-Marco R, Gómez-Ulla F, Mrejen S, Freund KB. Pachychoroid diseases of the macula. Med Hypothesis Discov Innov Ophthalmol. 2014;3(4):111-5.

107. Azar G, Wolff B, Mauget-Faÿsse M, Rispoli M, Savastano M-C, Lumbroso

B. Pachychoroid neovasculopathy: aspect on optical coherence tomography angiography. Acta Ophthalmologica. June 2017;95(4):421 -7.

108. Rebhun CB, Moult EM, Novais EA, Moreira-Neto C, Ploner SB, Louzada RN, et al. Polypoidal Choroidal Vasculopathy on Swept-Source Optical Coherence Tomography Angiography with Variable Interscan Time Analysis. Transl Vis Sci Technol. nov 2017;6(6):4.

109. Kim JY, Kwon OW, Oh HS, Kim SH, You YS. Optical coherence tomography angiography in patients with polypoidal choroidal vasculopathy. Graefe's Archive for Clinical and Experimental Ophthalmology. august 2016;254(8):1505-10.

110. Chi Y-T, Yang C-H, Cheng C-K. Optical Coherence Tomography Angiography for Assessment of the 3-Dimensional Structures of Polypoidal Choroidal Vasculopathy. JAMA Ophthalmology. Dec 1, 2017;135(12):1310.

111. Wang M, Zhou Y, Gao SS, Liu W, Huang Y, Huang D, et al. Evaluating Polypoidal Choroidal Vasculopathy With Optical Coherence Tomography Angiography. Invest Ophthalmol Vis Sci. Jul 2016;57(9):OCT526-32.

112. Seong S, Choo HG, Kim YJ, Kim JY, Lee JH, Oh HS, et al. Novel Findings of Polypoidal Choroidal Vasculopathy via Optical Coherence Tomography Angiography. Korean J Ophthalmol. Feb 2019;33(1):54-62.

113. Huang C-H, Yeh P-T, Hsieh Y-T, Ho T-C, Yang C-M, Yang C-H. Characterizing Branching Vascular Network Morphology in Polypoidal Choroidal Vasculopathy by Optical Coherence Tomography Angiography. Sci Rep [Internet]. 24 Jan. 2019 [cited 29 Apr. 2019];9. Available from: https://www.ncbi.nlm.nih.gov/pmc/articles/PMC6345899/

114. Tomiyasu T, Nozaki M, Yoshida M, Ogura Y. Characteristics of Polypoidal Choroidal Vasculopathy Evaluated by Optical Coherence Tomography Angiography. Invest Ophthalmol Vis Sci. 01 2016;57(9):OCT324-330.

115. Cheung CMG, Yanagi Y, Mohla A, Lee SY, Mathur R, Chan CM, et al. CHARACTERIZATION AND DIFFERENTIATION OF POLYPOIDAL CHOROIDAL VASCULOPATHY USING SWEPT SOURCE OPTICAL COHERENCE TOMOGRAPHY ANGIOGRAPHY. Retina (Philadelphia, Pa). august 2017;37(8):1464-74.

116. Polypoidal choroidal vasculopathy: a comprehensive clinical update [Internet]. [cited 29 Apr 2019]. Available from:

https://www.ncbi.nlm.nih.gov/pmc/articles/PMC6393826/

117. Srour M, Querques G, Semoun O, El Ameen A, Miere A, Sikorav A, et al. Optical coherence tomography angiography characteristics of polypoidal choroidal vasculopathy. Br J Ophthalmol. 2016;100(11):1489-93.

118. Teo KY, Yanagi Y, Lee S, Yeo IY, Tan GS, Mathur R, et al. COMPARISON OF OPTICAL COHERENCE TOMOGRAPHY ANGIOGRAPHIC CHANGES AFTER ANTI-VASCULAR ENDOTHELIAL GROWTH FACTOR THERAPY ALONE OR IN COMBINATION WITH PHOTODYNAMIC THERAPY IN POLYPOIDAL CHOROIDAL VASCULOPATHY. Retina. 1 Sep 2018;38(9):1675-87.

119. Chen G, Tzekov R, Li W, Jiang F, Mao S, Tong Y. Subfoveal Choroidal Thickness in Central Serous Chorioretinopathy: A Meta-Analysis. Cao C, editor. PLoS ONE. Jan 11, 2017;12(1):e0169152.

120. Cakir B, Reich M, Lang S, Bühler A, Ehlken C, Grundel B, et al. OCT Angiography of the Choriocapillaris in Central Serous Chorioretinopathy: A Quantitative Subgroup Analysis. Ophthalmol Ther. March 2019;8(1):75-86.

121. Kim YY, Flaxel CJ. Factors Influencing the Visual Acuity of Chronic Central Serous Chorioretinopathy. Korean J Ophthalmol. Apr 2011;25(2):90-7.

122. Spaide RF, Campeas L, Haas A, Yannuzzi LA, Fisher YL, Guyer DR, et al. Central Serous Chorioretinopathy in Younger and Older Adults. Ophthalmology. Dec 1, 1996;103(12):2070-80.

123. Peiretti E, Ferrara DC, Caminiti G, Mura M, Hughes J. Choroidal neovascularization in caucasian patients with longstanding central serous chorioretinopathy. Retina (Philadelphia, Pa). Jan 1, 2015;35(7):1360-7.

124. Factors Influencing the Visual Acuity of Chronic Central Serous Chorioretinopathy [Internet]. [cited 2020 May 17]. Available from: https://www.ncbi.nlm.nih.gov/pmc/articles/PMC3060399/

125. Daruich A, Matet A, Dirani A, Bousquet E, Zhao M, Farman N, et al. Central serous chorioretinopathy: Recent findings and new physiopathology hypothesis. Prog Retin Eye Res. Sept 2015;48:82-118.

126. Mrejen S, Spaide RF. Optical coherence tomography: imaging of the choroid and beyond. Surv Ophthalmol. Oct 2013;58(5):387-429.

127. Lai TYY, Wong RLM, Chan W-M. Long-Term Outcome of Half-Dose

Verteporfin Photodynamic Therapy for the Treatment of Central Serous Chorioretinopathy (An American Ophthalmological Society Thesis). Trans Am Ophthalmol Soc [Internet]. 2015 Sep [cited 2020 May 17]; 113. Available from: https://www.ncbi.nlm.nih.gov/pmc/articles/PMC4692328/

128. Toyama T, Ohtomo K, Noda Y, Ueta T. Polypoidal choroidal vasculopathy and history of central serous chorioretinopathy. Eye (Lond). August 2014;28(8):992-7.

129. Maggio E, Polito A, Freno MC, Pertile G. Multimodal imaging findings in a case of severe Central Serous Chorioretinopathy in an uncomplicated pregnancy. BMC Ophthalmology. 22 Dec 2015;15(1):183.

130. Matsumoto H, Kishi S, Sato T, Mukai R. Fundus autofluorescence of elongated photoreceptor outer segments in central serous chorioretinopathy. Am J Ophthalmol. Apr 2011;151(4):617-623.e1.

131. Manayath GJ, Ranjan R, Shah VS, Karandikar SS, Saravanan VR, Narendran V. Central serous chorioretinopathy: Current update on pathophysiology and multimodal imaging. Oman J Ophthalmol. 2018;11(2):103-12.

132. Spaide RF, Koizumi H, Pozzoni MC, Pozonni MC. Enhanced depth imaging spectral-domain optical coherence tomography. Am J Ophthalmol. Oct 2008;146(4):496-500.

133. Yang L, Jonas JB, Wei W. Optical coherence tomography-assisted enhanced depth imaging of central serous chorioretinopathy. Invest Ophthalmol Vis Sci. 12juill 2013;54(7):4659-65.

134. S. Mrejen, Author at Réalités Ophtalmologiques [Internet]. Réalités Ophtalmologiques. [cited May 17, 2020]. Available from: https://www.realites- ophtalmologiques.com/author/smrejen/

135. Piccolino FC, de La Longrais RR, Ravera G, Eandi CM, Ventre L, Abdollahi A, et al. The foveal photoreceptor layer and visual acuity loss in central serous chorioretinopathy. American Journal of Ophthalmology. Jan 1, 2005;139(1):87-99.

136. Costanzo E, Cohen SY, Miere A, Querques G, Capuano V, Semoun O, et al. Optical Coherence Tomography Angiography in Central Serous Chorioretinopathy. J Ophthalmol [Internet]. 2015 [cited 2019 May 1];2015. Available from: https://www.ncbi.nlm.nih.gov/pmc/articles/PMC4655052/

137. Chan SY, Wang Q, Wei WB, Jonas JB. OPTICAL COHERENCE

TOMOGRAPHIC ANGIOGRAPHY IN CENTRAL SEROUS CHORIORETINOPATHY: Retina. nov 2016;36(11):2051 -8.

138. De Bats F, Cornut P-L, Wolff B, Kodjikian L, Mauget-Faÿsse M. Dark and white lesions observed in central serous chorioretinopathy on optical coherence tomography angiography. European Journal of Ophthalmology. july 2018;28(4):446-53.

139. Shinojima A, Kawamura A, Mori R, Fujita K, Yuzawa M. Findings of Optical Coherence Tomographic Angiography at the Choriocapillaris Level in Central Serous Chorioretinopathy. Ophthalmologica. 2016;236(2):108-13.

140. Pichi F, Morara M, Veronese C, Ciardella AP. The overlapping spectrum of flat irregular pigment epithelial detachment investigated by optical coherence tomography angiography. International Ophthalmology. June 2018;38(3):975-83.

141. Matet A, Daruich A, Hardy S, Behar-Cohen F. PATTERNS OF CHORIOCAPILLARIS FLOW SIGNAL VOIDS IN CENTRAL SEROUS CHORIORETINOPATHY: An Optical Coherence Tomography Angiography Study. Retina (Philadelphia, Pa). nov 2019;39(11):2178-88.

142. Gawçcki M, Jaszczuk-Maciejewska A, Jurska-Jasko A, Kneba M, Grzybowski A.
Impairment of visual acuity and retinal morphology following resolved chronic central serous chorioretinopathy. BMC Ophthalmol [Internet]. 25 Jul. 2019 [cited 22 Mar. 2020]; 19. Available from: https://www.ncbi.nlm.nih.gov/pmc/articles/PMC6659242/

143. Xu Y, Su Y, Li L, Qi H, Zheng H, Chen C. Effect of Photodynamic Therapy on Optical Coherence Tomography Angiography in Eyes with Chronic Central Serous Chorioretinopathy. Ophthalmologica. 2017;237(3):167-72.

144. Filho MAB, de Carlo TE, Ferrara D, Adhi M, Baumal CR, Witkin AJ, et al. Association of Choroidal Neovascularization and Central Serous Chorioretinopathy With Optical Coherence Tomography Angiography. JAMA Ophthalmol. August 2015;133(8):899-906.

145. Hage R, Mrejen S, Krivosic V, Quentel G, Tadayoni R, Gaudric A. Flat Irregular Retinal Pigment Epithelium Detachments in Chronic Central Serous Chorioretinopathy and Choroidal Neovascularization. American Journal of Ophthalmology. May 1, 2015;159(5):890-903.e3.

146. Pang CE, Freund KB. Pachychoroid neovasculopathy. Retina (Philadelphia, Pa). jan 2015;35(1):1-9.

147. Bousquet E, Bonnin S, Mrejen S, Krivosic V, Tadayoni R, Gaudric A. OPTICAL COHERENCE TOMOGRAPHY ANGIOGRAPHY OF FLAT IRREGULAR PIGMENT EPITHELIUM DETACHMENT IN CHRONIC CENTRAL SEROUS CHORIORETINOPATHY: Retina. march 2018;38(3):629-38.

148. Bansal R, Dogra M, Mulkutkar S, Katoch D, Singh R, Gupta V, et al. Optical coherence tomography angiography versus fluorescein angiography in diagnosing choroidal neovascularization in chronic central serous chorioretinopathy. Indian J Ophthalmol. july 2019;67(7):1095 -100.

149. Quaranta-El Maftouhi M, El Maftouhi A, Eandi CM. Chronic central serous chorioretinopathy imaged by optical coherence tomographic angiography. Am J Ophthalmol. sept 2015;160(3):581-587.e1.

150. Flat irregular retinal pigment epithelium detachments in chronic central serous chorioretinopathy and choroidal neovascularization. [Internet]. [cited May 16, 2020]. Available from: https://reference.medscape.com/medline/abstract/25709063

151. Dansingani KK, Balaratnasingam C, Klufas MA, Sarraf D, Freund KB. Optical Coherence Tomography Angiography of Shallow Irregular Pigment Epithelial Detachments In Pachychoroid Spectrum Disease. Am J Ophthalmol. dec 2015;160(6):1243-1254.e2.

152. Gruber M, Wolf J, Stahl A, Ness T, Scholl H, Agostini H, et al. Novel insights into retinal neovascularization secondary to central serous chorioretinopathy using 3D optical coherence tomography angiography. Am J Ophthalmol Case Rep [Internet].
Feb 11, 2020 [cited May 8, 2020];18. Available from: https://www.ncbi.nlm.nih.gov/pmc/articles/PMC7036447/

153. Pierru A, Girmens J-F, Héron E, Paques M. Retinal venous occlusions. Journal Français d'Ophtalmologie. oct 2017;40(8):696-705.

154. Coscas F, Glacet-Bernard A, Miere A, Caillaux V, Uzzan J, Lupidi M, et al. Optical Coherence Tomography Angiography in Retinal Vein Occlusion: Evaluation of Superficial and Deep Capillary Plexa. American Journal of Ophthalmology. jan 2016;161:160-171.e2.

155. Spaide RF. RETINAL VASCULAR CYSTOID MACULAR EDEMA: Review and New Theory. Retina (Philadelphia, Pa). oct 2016;36(10):1823-42.

156. Spaide RF. PERIPHERAL AREAS OF NONPERFUSION IN TREATED CENTRAL RETINAL VEIN OCCLUSION AS IMAGED BY WIDE-FIELD FLUORESCEIN ANGIOGRAPHY. RETINA. May

2011;31(5):829-837.

157. al BM et. [Analysis of changes in central macular thickness based on optical coherence tomography angiography findings in retinal vein occlusion]. - PubMed - NCBI [Internet]. [cited 8 Apr 2019]. Available from: https://www.ncbi.nlm.nih.gov/pubmed/27911421

158. Ang M, Tan A, Cheung CMG, Keane P, Dolz-Marco R, Sng C, et al. Optical coherence tomography angiography: a review of current and future clinical applications. Graefe's Archive for Clinical and Experimental Ophthalmology. 9 Jan 2018;256.

159. Khan HA, Mehmood A, Khan QA, Iqbal F, Rasheed F, Khan N, et al. A major review of optical coherence tomography angiography. Expert Review of Ophthalmology. 3 Sep 2017;12(5):373-85.

160. Kang J-W, Yoo R, Jo YH, Kim HC. CORRELATION OF MICROVASCULAR STRUCTURES ON OPTICAL COHERENCE TOMOGRAPHY ANGIOGRAPHY WITH VISUAL ACUITY IN RETINAL VEIN OCCLUSION. Retina (Philadelphia, Pa). sept 2017;37(9):1700-9.

161. Wons J, Pfau M, Wirth MA, Freiberg FJ, Becker MD, Michels S. Optical Coherence Tomography Angiography of the Foveal Avascular Zone in Retinal Vein Occlusion. Ophthalmologica. 2016;235(4):195 -202.

162. Casselholmde Salles M, Kvanta A, Amrén U, Epstein D. Optical Coherence Tomography Angiography in Central Retinal Vein Occlusion: Correlation Between the Foveal Avascular Zone and Visual Acuity. Investigative Ophthalmology & Visual Science. 13 Jul 2016;57(9):OCT242.

163. Costanzo E, Parravano M, Gilardi M, Cavalleri M, Sacconi R, Aragona E, et al. Retinal and Choroidal Microvascular Changes in Retinal Vein Occlusion Analyzed by Two Different Optical Coherence Tomography Angiography Devices. Ophthalmologica. Feb 5, 2019;1-8.

164. Schmidt-Erfurth U, Garcia-Arumi J, Gerendas BS, Midena E, Sivaprasad S, Tadayoni R, et al. Guidelines for the Management of Retinal Vein Occlusion by the European Society of Retina Specialists (EURETINA). Ophthalmologica. 2019;242(3):123-62.

165. Seknazi D, Coscas F, Sellam A, Rouimi F, Coscas G, Souied EH, et al. OPTICAL COHERENCE TOMOGRAPHY ANGIOGRAPHY IN RETINAL VEIN OCCLUSION: Correlations Between Macular Vascular Density, Visual Acuity, and Peripheral Nonperfusion Area on Fluorescein Angiography. Retina (Philadelphia, Pa). 2018;38(8):1562-70.

166. Glacet-Bernard A, Sellam A, Coscas F, Coscas G, Souied EH. Optical coherence tomography angiography in retinal vein occlusion treated with dexamethasone implant: a new test for follow-up evaluation. Eur J Ophthalmol. August 4, 2016;26(5):460-8.

167. Sellam A, Glacet-Bernard A, Coscas F, Miere A, Coscas G, Souied EH. QUALITATIVE AND QUANTITATIVE FOLLOW-UP USING OPTICAL COHERENCE TOMOGRAPHY ANGIOGRAPHY OF RETINAL VEIN OCCLUSION TREATED WITH ANTI-VEGF: Optical Coherence Tomography Angiography Follow-up of Retinal Vein Occlusion. Retina. June 2017;37(6):1176-84.

168. Suzuki N, Hirano Y, Tomiyasu T, Kurobe R, Yasuda Y, Esaki Y, et al. Collateral vessels on optical coherence tomography angiography in eyes with branch retinal vein occlusion. Br J Ophthalmol. 22 Nov 2018;

169. Suzuki N, Hirano Y, Tomiyasu T, Esaki Y, Uemura A, Yasukawa T, et al. Retinal Hemodynamics Seen on Optical Coherence Tomography Angiography Before and After Treatment of Retinal Vein Occlusion. Invest Ophthalmol Vis Sci. 1 Oct 2016;57(13):5681-7.

170. Kimura M, Nozaki M, Yoshida M, Ogura Y. Wide-field optical coherence tomography angiography using extended field imaging technique to evaluate the nonperfusion area in retinal vein occlusion. Clinical Ophthalmology. july 2016;Volume 10:1291-5.

171. Shiraki A, Sakimoto S, Tsuboi K, Wakabayashi T, Hara C, Fukushima Y, et al. Evaluation of retinal nonperfusion in branch retinal vein occlusion using wide-field optical coherence tomography angiography. Acta Ophthalmol. sept 2019;97(6):e913-8.

172. Fukutomi A, Tsuboi K, Ono H, Ishida Y, Kamei M. Sequential Observations of Conversion from Nonischemic to Ischemic Central Retinal Vein Occlusion Using Optical Coherence Tomography Angiography. Case Rep Ophthalmol Med. 2018;2018:1354217.

173. Sellam A, Glacet-Bernard A, Coscas F, Souied EH. Retinal arterial perfusion disorder and optical coherence tomography-angiography. Journal Français d'Ophtalmologie. may 2017;40(5):353-62.

174. Abdellah MM. Multimodal Imaging of Acute Central Retinal Artery Occlusion. Med Hypothesis Discov Innov Ophthalmol. 2019;8(4):283 -90.

175. Wang X, Sun B, Wang J, Jia Y, Huang D, Dong J. Quantitative evaluation of retinal artery occlusion using optical coherence tomography angiography. Medicine (Baltimore) [Internet]. 5 Oct 2018 [cited 5 Apr 2020];97(40). Available from:

https://www.ncbi.nlm.nih.gov/pmc/articles/PMC6200535/

176. Yang S, Liu X, Li H, Xu J, Wang F. Optical coherence tomography angiography characteristics of acute retinal arterial occlusion. BMC Ophthalmol [Internet]. Jul 10, 2019 [cited Feb 18, 2020];19. Available from: https://www.ncbi.nlm.nih.gov/pmc/articles/PMC6621973/

177. Baumal CR. Optical Coherence Tomography Angiography of Retinal Artery Occlusion. In: Bandello F, Souied EH, Querques G, editors. Developments in Ophthalmology [Internet]. S. Karger AG; 2016 [cited 26 Jul 2019]. p. 122-31. Available from: https://www.karger.com/Article/FullText/442803

178. Bonnin S, Krivosic V, Cognat E, Tadayoni R. Visibility of Blood Flow on Optical Coherence Tomography Angiography in a Case of Branch Retinal Artery Occlusion. J Ophthalmic Vis Res. 2018;13(1):75-7.

179. Çelik T, Bilen F, Yalçindag FN, Atilla H. Optical Coherence Tomography Angiography in Branch Retinal Artery Occlusion. Turk J Ophthalmol. June 2018;48(3):150-4.

180. Lee AY, Zhang Q, Baughman DM, Mudumbai R, Wang RK, Lee CS. Evaluation of bilateral central retinal artery occlusions with optical coherence tomography-based microangiography: a case report. Journal of Medical Case Reports [Internet]. 2016 [cited 22 Apr 2019]; 10. Available from: https://www.ncbi.nlm.nih.gov/pmc/articles/PMC5090894/

181. Philippakis E, Dupas B, Bonnin P, Hage R, Gaudric A, Tadayoni R. OPTICAL COHERENCE TOMOGRAPHY ANGIOGRAPHY SHOWS DEEP CAPILLARY PLEXUS HYPOPERFUSION IN INCOMPLETE CENTRAL RETINAL ARTERY OCCLUSION. Retinal Cases & Brief Reports. oct 2015;9(4):333-8.

182. Sellam A, Glacet-Bernard A, Coscas F, Souied EH. [Abnormal retinal artery perfusion and optical coherence tomography angiography]. J Fr Ophthalmol. May 2017;40(5):353-62.

183. de Castro-Abeger AH, de Carlo TE, Duker JS, Baumal CR. Optical Coherence Tomography Angiography Compared to Fluorescein Angiography in Branch Retinal Artery Occlusion. Ophthalmic Surg Lasers Imaging Retina. dec 2015;46(10):1052-4.

184. Wu S-C, Villegas VM, Kovach JL. Optical Coherence Tomography Angiography of Combined Central Retinal Artery and Vein Occlusion. Case Rep Ophthalmol Med. 2018;2018:4342158.

185. Corbelli E, Carnevali A, Marchese A, Cicinelli MV, Querques L, Sacconi R, et al. OPTICAL COHERENCE TOMOGRAPHY ANGIOGRAPHY FEATURES OF ANGIOID STREAKS: Retina. sept 2017;1.

186. Marchese A, Parravano M, Rabiolo A, Carnevali A, Corbelli E, Cicinelli MV, et al. Optical coherence tomography analysis of evolution of Bruch's membrane features in angioid streaks. Eye. nov 2017;31(11):1600-5.

187. Mentes J, Karaca I, Sermet F. Multimodal imaging characteristics of quiescent type 1 neovascularization in an eye with angioid streaks. American Journal of Ophthalmology Case Reports. june 2018;10:132-6.

188. Stanga PE, Papayannis A, Tsamis E, Chwiejczak K, Stringa F, Jalil A, et al. Swept- Source Optical Coherence Tomography Angiography of Paediatric Macular Diseases. In: Bandello F, Souied EH, Querques G, editors. Developments in Ophthalmology [Internet]. S. Karger AG; 2016 [cited 2019 May 2]. p. 166-73. Available from: https://www.karger.com/Article/FullText/442809

189. Treder M, Lauermann JL, Alnawaiseh M, Heiduschka P, Eter N. Quantitative changes in flow density in patients with adult-onset foveomacular vitelliform dystrophy: an OCT angiography study. Graefe's Archive for Clinical and Experimental Ophthalmology. jan 2018;256(1):23-8.

190. Qian CX, Charran D, Strong CR, Steffens TJ, Jayasundera T, Heckenlively JR. Optical Coherence Tomography Examination of the Retinal Pigment Epithelium in Best Vitelliform Macular Dystrophy. Ophthalmology. apr 2017;124(4):456-63.

191. Dansingani KK, Tan ACS, Gilani F, Phasukkijwatana N, Novais E, Querques L, et al. Subretinal Hyperreflective Material Imaged With Optical Coherence Tomography Angiography. American Journal of Ophthalmology. sept 2016;169:235-48.

192. Joshi KM, Nesper PL, Fawzi AA, Mirza RG. OPTICAL COHERENCE TOMOGRAPHY ANGIOGRAPHY IN ADULT-ONSET FOVEOMACULAR VITELLIFORM DYSTROPHY. 2017;0(0):6.

193. Guduru A, Gupta A, Tyagi M, Jalali S, Chhablani J. Optical coherence tomography angiography characterisation of Best disease and associated choroidal neovascularisation. British Journal of Ophthalmology. August 1, 2017;bjophthalmol- 2017-310586.

194. Stattin M, Ahmed D, Glittenberg C, Krebs I, Ansari-Shahrezaei S. OPTICAL COHERENCE TOMOGRAPHY ANGIOGRAPHY FOR THE DETECTION OF SECONDARY CHOROIDAL

NEOVASCULARIZATION IN VITELLIFORM MACULAR DYSTROPHY: Retinal Cases & Brief Reports. august 2017;1.

195. Jia Y, Bailey ST, Hwang TS, McClintic SM, Gao SS, Pennesi ME, et al. Quantitative optical coherence tomography angiography of vascular abnormalities in the living human eye. Proc Natl Acad Sci U S A. May 5, 2015;112(18):E2395-402.

196. Mastropasqua R, Di Antonio L, Di Staso S, Agnifili L, Di Gregorio A, Ciancaglini M, et al. Optical Coherence Tomography Angiography in Retinal Vascular Diseases and Choroidal Neovascularization. J Ophthalmol [Internet]. 2015 [cited 5 Jul 2019];2015. Available from: https://www.ncbi.nlm.nih.gov/pmc/articles/PMC4600507/

197. Miyata M, Ooto S, Hata M, Yamashiro K, Tamura H, Akagi-Kurashige Y, et al. Detection of Myopic Choroidal Neovascularization Using Optical Coherence Tomography Angiography. Am J Ophthalmol. May 2016;165:108-14.

198. Querques L, Giuffrè C, Corvi F, Zucchiatti I, Carnevali A, Vitis LAD, et al. Optical coherence tomography angiography of myopic choroidal neovascularisation. British Journal of Ophthalmology. May 1, 2017;101(5):609-15.

199. Bagchi A, Schwartz R, Hykin P, Sivaprasad S. Diagnostic algorithm utilising multimodal imaging including optical coherence tomography angiography for the detection of myopic choroidal neovascularisation. Eye [Internet]. 26 Feb 2019 [cited 7 May 2019]; Available from: http://www.nature.com/articles/s41433-019-0378-2

200. Bruyère E, Miere A, Cohen S, Martiano D, Sikorav A, Popeanga A, et al. NEOVASCULARIZATION SECONDARY TO HIGH MYOPIA IMAGED BY OPTICAL COHERENCE TOMOGRAPHY ANGIOGRAPHY. Retina. 1 Nov 2017;37(11):2095-101.

201. Cennamo G, Amoroso F, Schiemer S, Velotti N, Alfieri M, de Crecchio G. Optical coherence tomography angiography in myopic choroidal neovascularization after intravitreal ranibizumab. Eur J Ophthalmol. March 2019;29(2):239-43.

202. Kuehlewein L, Sadda SR, Sarraf D. OCT angiography and sequential quantitative analysis of type 2 neovascularization after ranibizumab therapy. Eye (Lond). july 2015;29(7):932-5.

203. Al-Sheikh M, Phasukkijwatana N, Dolz-Marco R, Rahimi M, Iafe NA, Freund KB, et al. Quantitative OCT Angiography of the Retinal

Microvasculature and the Choriocapillaris in Myopic Eyes. Invest Ophthalmol Vis Sci. 01 2017;58(4):2063-9.

204. Kumar A, Vohra R, Agrawal S, Chawla R, Azad SV, Venkatesh P, et al. Characterization of Idiopathic Choroidal Neovascularization Using Fluorescein Angiography, Indocyanine Green Angiography, and Optical Coherence Tomography Angiography. Ophthalmic Surg Lasers Imaging Retina. 01 2018;49(7):516-22.

205. Chen Q, Yu X, Sun Z, Dai H. The Application of OCTA in Assessment of Anti- VEGF Therapy for Idiopathic Choroidal Neovascularization. J Ophthalmol [Internet]. 2016 [cited 5 Jul 2019];2016. Available from: https://www.ncbi.nlm.nih.gov/pmc/articles/PMC4947658/

206. Moussa M, Leila M, Khalid H. Imaging choroidal neovascular membrane using en face swept-source optical coherence tomography angiography. Clin Ophthalmol. 2017;11:1859-69.

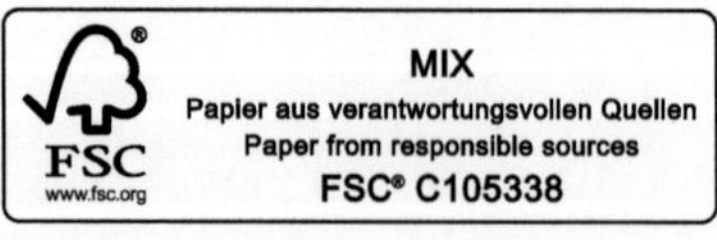

Printed by Books on Demand GmbH, Norderstedt / Germany